Cognitive-Behavioral Treatment of Obesity

Cognitive-Behavioral Treatment of Obesity

A CLINICIAN'S GUIDE

Zafra Cooper

Christopher G. Fairburn

Deborah M. Hawker

THE GUILFORD PRESS

New York   London

© 2003 The Guilford Press

A Division of Guilford Publications, Inc.

72 Spring Street, New York, NY 10012

www.guilford.com

Printed in the United States of America

This book is printed on acid-free paper.

Last digit is print number: 9 8 7 6 5 4 3 2 1

Library of Congress Cataloging-in-Publication Data

Cooper, Zafra.
  Cognitive-behavioral treatment of obesity : a clinician's guide /
Zafra Cooper, Christopher G. Fairburn, Deborah M. Hawker.
      p. cm.
Includes bibliographical references and index.
    ISBN 1-57230-888-5
  1. Obesity—Treatment. 2. Cognitive therapy. I. Fairburn,
Christopher G. II. Hawker, Deborah M. III. Title.
RC552.O25 C66 2003
616.3'9806–dc21   2002154655

About the Authors

Zafra Cooper DPhil, DipClinPsych, is Principal Research Psychologist and Honorary Senior Clinical Lecturer in Psychiatry at the University of Oxford. She has a background in both psychology and philosophy, having completed her graduate work in the philosophy of mind. Dr. Cooper has conducted research on the role of social factors in the persistence of depression, focusing particularly on the role of life events. Her specialized research interests are the nature and treatment of eating disorders and obesity. She has been involved in studies of the etiology, course, and assessment of eating disorders, and in developing and evaluating cognitive-behavioral treatments for eating disorders and obesity. Dr. Cooper has held research grants and has published in the area.

Christopher G. Fairburn, DM, FRCPsych, FMedSci, is Wellcome Principal Research Fellow and Professor of Psychiatry at the University of Oxford. He specializes in research on the nature and treatment of eating disorders and obesity. His studies have addressed many aspects of eating disorders, including their diagnostic status, epidemiology, etiology, assessment, course, and treatment. Professor Fairburn has a particular interest in the development and evaluation of psychological treatments. He has held research grants in Great Britain and the United States, and he has published extensively in the area. Professor Fairburn has twice been a fellow at the Center for Advanced Study in the Behavioral Sciences at Stanford University. He is a Fellow of the Academy of Medical Sciences.

Deborah M. Hawker, PhD, DClinPsy, is Research Psychologist and Honorary Principal Clinical Psychologist in the Department of Psychiatry at the University of Oxford. She has worked as a therapist in studies evaluating cognitive-behavioral treatments for eating disorders and obesity, and has conducted cross-cultural research on eating disorders and on bereavement reactions. She is on the executive committee of the United Kingdom national charity Anorexia and Bulimia Care. Dr. Hawker also specializes in working with overseas aid workers, mainly addressing issues related to depression, anxiety disorders, and chronic fatigue syndrome. She is the author of three books.

Preface

This book describes a cognitive-behavioral treatment for obesity together with an outline of the theory on which it is based. The treatment is described in detail in the form of a clinician's manual. It includes information on how to help patients lose weight, increase their activity level, and address concerns about shape and weight. Particular emphasis is placed on helping patients maintain their new lower weight. The treatment is primarily intended for patients with a body mass index (BMI)[1] between 30 and 40 (i.e., those with obesity), but it is also relevant to those with lesser degrees of excess weight (i.e., those whose BMI is between 25 and 30). We do not have experience using the treatment with patients whose BMI is over 40, although it is likely that elements of it may be useful in combination with other approaches.

We have written this book in response to requests from clinicians for guidance as to how to treat patients using this cognitive-behavioral approach. These requests reflect the absence of detailed clinical guidelines of this type. In some respects, this book is premature as we do not yet have research evidence to support the long-term effectiveness of the treatment or data on the theory on which it is based. We recognize the need for such evidence and are nearing the completion of an evaluation of the treatment in a long-term randomized controlled trial (hereafter termed the "Oxford study"). Nevertheless, we have chosen to publish this manual before the study has been finished because, even in the absence of such data, we believe that there is a clinical need for guidelines of the type that it provides.

Our background is in the field of eating disorders. It was through our work on the treatment of eating disorders that we became aware that some of the problems that are successfully addressed in the context of treating bulimia nervosa and anorexia nervosa are also relevant to patients with obesity. Our experience in successfully treating, with cognitive-behavioral therapy, problems such

---

[1]Body mass index is weight in kilograms divided by height in meters squared—that is, (weight in kg)/(height in m^2).

as binge eating, dissatisfaction with body shape and weight, and issues concerning control over eating led us to believe that similar principles might be applied to the treatment of obesity. We were also aware that there were problems with existing treatments for obesity, particularly that of weight regain following successful weight loss. Within this context and on the basis of detailed clinical observations, we developed a theory of the psychological processes involved in weight regain (Cooper & Fairburn, 2001, 2002). This in turn led to the gradual development of the treatment described in this book, which is, with some minor modifications, the treatment being evaluated in the Oxford study.

This book has been written for professionals from any discipline who treat patients with obesity or those with problems of long-term weight control. When implementing this cognitive-behavioral treatment, we believe that it is important to follow the principles specified. In the book we have described the treatment much as we have used it in the Oxford study, but we recommend that clinicians use the treatment flexibly according to their own and their patients' circumstances. For example, the treatment could be adapted for use with groups of patients rather than on a one-to-one basis as we have used it, and clinicians may wish to vary the number of sessions or the duration of treatment.

In describing the treatment, we have tried to keep references to the clinical and research literature to a minimum so as to present the material in a way that is easy to read and most useful for therapists wanting to implement the treatment. Where we have included references, we have tried as far as possible to confine them to one authoritative text, *Eating Disorders and Obesity: A Comprehensive Handbook* (Fairburn & Brownell, 2002), as the book contains many relevant summary chapters written by experts in the field, each of which provides specific guidelines for further reading. By having done this we hope that we have provided readers with good sources of further information without their having to pursue large numbers of individual references.

As obesity is a medical condition and we work within a hospital, we have used the term *patient* to refer to those receiving the treatment described. We recognize that some people prefer the term *client*, and we regard this term as equally acceptable. By using *patient* we do not intend to imply that the person with obesity is a passive recipient of the treatment—far from it. As we emphasize in the book, and in common with all cognitive-behavioral treatments, treatment should be an intensely collaborative process with the clinician and patient working together to help the patient overcome his or her problems.

Acknowledgments

All three authors are supported by the Wellcome Trust: CGF is supported by a Principal Research Fellowship (046386), and ZC and DMH are supported by a program grant (046386). The Oxford study is also supported by the Wellcome Trust. Without the Wellcome Trust's sustained support over many years, this work would not have been possible.

We want to highlight and acknowledge the contributions of three of our Oxford colleagues. Gillie Bonner was responsible for developing many of the dietary elements of the treatment. She also assembled and edited most of the clinical vignettes and was a therapist in the Oxford study. Liz Eeley also contributed significantly to the dietary components of the treatment. Susan Byrne is involved in ongoing tests of the cognitive-behavioral theory on which the treatment is based, and she also was a therapist in the Oxford study.

Finally, we want to thank the following experts in the obesity field for their support and encouragement: John E. Blundell, Kelly D. Brownell, Nick Finer, Susan A. Jebb, Thomas A. Wadden, G. Terence Wilson, Rena R. Wing, and Michael G. Perri.

Contents

Cognitive-Behavioral Treatment of Obesity

CHAPTER 1

Introduction

In principle, weight control is simple.[1] It requires balancing energy input and energy expenditure over the long term. For many people this requires little or no conscious effort. It happens by default. However, the steady rise in the prevalence of people who are overweight or obese indicates that there are increasing numbers of people of all ages for whom weight control is less straightforward. The explanation for this rise is debated but it is likely to stem from both an increase in energy intake (i.e., eating and drinking to excess) and a decrease in energy expenditure (i.e., being underactive). To counter this phenomenon people need to be both educated about the processes involved in successful long-term weight control and helped to apply them.

The treatment described in this manual is a new cognitive-behavioral treatment for obesity. The treatment is primarily intended for patients with a body mass index (BMI[2]) between 30 and 40, but it is also relevant for those whose BMI is between 25 and 30. We do not have experience using it with patients whose BMI is above 40, but it is likely that some aspects of it may be useful in combination with other approaches. The treatment was designed to be applied on a one-to-one basis and a major focus is on the problem of posttreatment weight regain, which is arguably the most pressing issue in the treatment of obesity.

In this chapter we describe in principle the defining features of cognitive-behavioral therapy and how it differs from behavior therapy. After a brief review of the literature on the use of these treatments to help people with obesity, we highlight the clinical problem of posttreatment weight regain.

---

[1] This chapter and the following one are edited and updated versions of Cooper and Fairburn (2002). Copyright 2002 by The Guilford Press. Adapted with permission.

[2] Body mass index is weight in kilograms divided by height in meters squared—that is, (weight in kg) / (height in m^2).

1

The Characteristics of Cognitive-Behavioral Therapy

Cognitive-behavioral treatments have three features, which together distinguish them from behavioral therapy and from other forms of psychological treatment.

1. *Cognitive-behavioral treatments are based on a cognitive conceptualization of the processes that maintain the problem in question.* In other words, these treatments are derived from a theory concerning the maintenance of the problem that assigns central importance to the contribution of cognitive processes. For example, in the case of depression, it is proposed that the disorder is maintained to a large extent by the presence of certain characteristic depressive thoughts and assumptions regarding the self, the world, and the future (Beck, 1976); in bulimia nervosa, it is proposed that a central maintaining mechanism is the judging of self-worth largely in terms of shape or weight (Fairburn, 1985); and in panic disorder, it is proposed that the key psychopathological feature is the interpretation of bodily sensations as being highly threatening (Clark, 1986). In each of these disorders, the particular cognitive theory of maintenance provides the basis for a specific cognitive-behavioral treatment.

2. *Cognitive-behavioral treatments are designed to modify the postulated cognitive and behavioral maintaining mechanisms, the prediction being that this is necessary for there to be lasting change.* A major aim of cognitive-behavioral treatments is to produce change in the central cognitive processes that maintain the disorder, although other features are also directly addressed. Thus, for example, in depression a key aspect of treatment is to modify depressive thoughts about the self and the world; in the case of bulimia nervosa, treatment aims to change the central importance assigned to shape and weight in the judgment of self-worth; and in panic disorder, the aim is to alter patients' interpretation of their bodily sensations. Examples of the other features addressed include the social withdrawal seen in depression, the characteristically rigid and extreme dieting of many patients with eating disorders, and the avoidance of fear-engendering situations found in anxiety disorders.

3. *Cognitive-behavioral treatments use a combination of cognitive and behavioral procedures to help the patient identify and change the targeted maintaining mechanisms.* Commonly used treatment procedures include the presentation and personalization of the relevant cognitive theory of maintenance; the use of behavioral "experiments" to help patients try new ways of behaving, and to help them test their expectations regarding the consequences of behavior change; and the systematic identification and evaluation of dysfunctional thoughts and assumptions.

In many other respects cognitive-behavioral therapy is similar to behavior therapy. Many therapeutic techniques are common to both treatments. Both are short-term, problem-oriented treatments, and both are primarily focused on the present and future rather than on the past. Both involve the presentation of an explicit model of the maintenance of the problem in question; both use a similar collaborative therapeutic style; and both require patients to be active participants in the change process. Lastly, both are committed to seeking empirical evidence to evaluate their effectiveness and to evolving in response to clinical and research findings. Despite these similarities, cognitive-behavioral therapy, unlike behavior therapy, stresses cognitive processes. The primary aim of cognitive-behavioral therapy is to produce cognitive change; and behavioral experiments and cognitive restructuring are central characteristics.

Cognitive-Behavioral Therapy and Obesity

There is a substantial body of evidence supporting the use of behavior therapy in the treatment of obesity (Wilson & Brownell, 2002; Wing, 1998, 2002). It reliably results in an average weight loss of about 10% of initial weight (among treatment completers), a weight loss that is thought to result in clinically significant health benefits (Blackburn, 2002; Goldstein, 1992; Kanders & Blackburn, 1992; Tremblay et al., 1999; Wing & Jeffrey, 1995), as well as psychological benefit (Foster & Wadden, 2002; Seidell & Tijhuis, 2002). Equally reliably, however, the lost weight is regained over the following 3 years (Jeffery et al., 2000; Perri, 1998, 2002; Wilson & Brownell, 2002).

Behavioral treatments for obesity have evolved since the 1960s when they were first developed. Among the developments has been the addition of cognitive procedures and, sometimes, this has resulted in the relabeling of the treatment as "cognitive-behavioral therapy" (e.g., DeLucia & Kalodner, 1990; Foreyt & Poston, 1998; Kalodner & DeLucia, 1991; Kirsch, Montgomery, & Sapirstein, 1995). Nowadays many behavioral treatments include treatment sessions on topics such as negative thinking and relapse prevention (e.g., Wardle & Rapoport, 1998), but this occurs in the context of the general characteristics of a behavioral treatment for obesity. As described by Wing (1998, pp. 860–862), these characteristics are:

- It is delivered to groups of 10–20 patients.
- The treatment is presented as a series of preplanned "lessons." The entire group receives lesson 1 on week 1, lesson 2 on week 2, and so on.
- There is no assessment of whether the lessons relate to individual participants' particular problems or whether participants have mastered the contents of any one lesson before moving on to the next. On the other hand, many of these treatments include training in problem solving, which does provide participants with a general strategy for addressing their particular difficulties.
- Many programs use a team of therapists (e.g., a behavioral therapist, an exercise physiologist, and a nutritionist) and rotate therapists by topic.
- Treatment usually involves weekly meetings for 16–24 weeks with a series of less frequent meetings thereafter.
- The principal content of such treatments is the self-monitoring of eating; the setting of specific behavioral goals regarding eating and exercise;

lessons on nutrition; emphasis on increasing both lifestyle activity and formal exercise; the use of stimulus control techniques; training in problem solving; simple cognitive restructuring; and relapse prevention (see Wadden & Osei, 2002).

Such treatments bear almost no resemblance to cognitive-behavioral therapy in their theoretical basis (which, if present, places little weight on the contribution of cognitive processes), aims (which are to change eating and exercise habits rather than to also achieve cognitive change), or treatment procedures (which are almost exclusively behavioral). Indeed, their highly structured prescriptive format bears only a limited resemblance to behavior therapy as commonly practiced outside the treatment of obesity. Rather, these treatments might better be characterized as behaviorally oriented group psychoeducational interventions. However, it must be acknowledged that there is no evidence that a more flexible and individualized form of behavior treatment would be any more effective.

To our knowledge no cognitive-behavioral theories or treatments for obesity (as defined above) have been described or evaluated. Cognitive-behavioral treatments have been developed for problems associated with obesity such as binge eating (Fairburn, Marcus, & Wilson, 1993) and body image disturbance (Rosen, 1997), and there are cognitive-behavioral "nondieting" treatments which discourage calorie restriction in order to lose weight and aim instead to promote healthy eating, to improve participants' well-being, and to encourage physical activity (e.g., Rapoport, Clark, & Wardle, 2000; Sbrocco, Nedegaard, Stone, & Lewis, 1999; Tanco, Linden, & Earle, 1998). In none of these treatments is the primary emphasis on achieving weight loss or on preventing weight regain, although it is clearly recognized that changes in weight might occur as a result of treatment.

The Problem of Weight Regain

It has recently been written that "The maintenance of treatment effects represents the single greatest challenge in the long-term management of obesity" (Perri, 1998, p. 526). This widely held view is based on a substantial body of evidence indicating that a weight loss of 5–10% can be achieved with both behavioral and pharmacological treatments for obesity and that this loss is probably worth achieving from the standpoint of physical health. The problem is that once treatment is stopped, the lost weight is regained.

Two forms of long-term treatment for the prevention of weight regain have been advocated. The first is long-term drug treatment (see Aronne, 2002). For a number of reasons, this is not likely to be a complete answer. First, many patients would prefer not to be treated with drugs and, as treatment is extended in duration, there are likely to be increasing problems with the acceptability of drug treatment and therefore compliance. Second, there is the ever-present possibility that long-term drug use will be associated with adverse physical effects.[3] Third, there are situations in which drug treatment would be inappropriate, for example, during pregnancy.

The second approach advocated is long-term, or even indefinite, psychological or behavioral treatment. This is supported by evidence that suggests that extending treatment delays weight regain (Perri, 1998, 2002; Perri, McKelvey, Renjilian, Nezu, Shermer, & Viegener, 2001); evidence that intensive long-term treatment (involving rapid and vigorous response to signs of relapse) can be effective (Bjorvell & Rosner, 1992); and evidence that some people benefit from long-term group pressure and support (Latner, Stunkard, Wilson, Jackson, Zelitch, & Labouvie, 2000). However, this evidence rests largely on an "efficacy" perspective in which the focus has been on the outcome of the (often small) subgroup of participants who both accept and comply with these types of long-term treatment (Jeffery et al., 2000). Moreover, the majority of studies of extended (rather than indefinite) treatment have not reported sufficient follow-up data to demonstrate that the familiar trend toward weight regain does not occur after the end of the extended treatment period. Thus, the true clinical utility of long-term treatment remains to be established.

---

[3] Salutary in this regard is the association between valvular heart disease and the use of the antiobesity drugs fenfluramine, dexfenfluramine, and phentermine (Connolly et al., 1997; Ryan et al., 1999). It took many years for this association to come to light.

CHAPTER 2

An Overview of the Theory and Treatment

We suggest that the disappointing long-term results of behavioral treatments for obesity may be attributed, in part, to two factors: first, the neglect of the contribution of cognitive factors to weight regain; and second, the ambiguity over treatment goals that is often present in long-term treatment programs—that is, the lack of a clear distinction between the objective of achieving *weight loss* (which requires sustaining an energy deficit), and the objective of maintaining the *weight lost* (i.e., maintaining the new lower weight). Accordingly, we have developed a different therapeutic approach to the prevention of post-treatment weight regain. This is derived from a cognitive-behavioral analysis of the processes responsible for weight regain, and it involves directing treatment at these processes.

A full account of our cognitive-behavioral analysis of weight regain is presented elsewhere (Cooper & Fairburn, 2001). Briefly, we suggest that weight regain is due to failure to engage in effective weight-control behavior, and that this, in turn, is a result of two interrelated processes. The first is a progressive decrease in patients' belief that they can control their weight to a worthwhile extent. This is in response to the decline in the rate of weight loss experienced by most patients after 4–6 months of attempting to lose weight, and the growing realization that they will achieve neither their weight loss goals nor the other objectives that they had hoped to achieve as a result of losing weight. These other objectives (which we term *primary goals*) commonly include a desire to improve appearance (particularly to modify shape), a desire to improve self-confidence and self-respect, a desire to be more active, and a desire to improve health. We suggest that the realization that they will not achieve the weight loss they had hoped for, nor the other benefits that they thought would result, eventually leads them to believe that their attempts to control their weight are not worth the considerable effort. As a result they abandon their striving for further weight loss.

Under these circumstances, the second postulated process begins to operate; that is, the abandoning of weight control altogether and a return to prior eating habits, with the result that a positive energy balance develops. This response is paradoxical, as it would seem more rational for patients to wish to maintain whatever benefits they have obtained, even if these are less than those originally sought. We suggest that patients do not do this because they are not in the right frame of mind to even consider, let alone accept, weight maintenance as a worthwhile goal. This is because they undervalue the weight loss they have achieved, and they tend to neglect, minimize, or discount any other gains that have resulted (in terms of achieving their primary goals). As a consequence they underestimate the extent to which they are already controlling their weight. In addition, the conflating by patients (and their therapists) of the processes of weight loss and weight maintenance results in their failing to appreciate the distinctiveness of weight maintenance and as a result their neglecting the importance of acquiring and practicing effective weight maintenance skills (as distinct from those required for weight loss).

The New Cognitive-Behavioral Treatment

On the basis of this cognitive-behavioral analysis, we developed the treatment described in this book.[1] The treatment is designed not only to achieve weight loss but also to minimize subsequent weight regain. To achieve the latter objective, the treatment is directed at the various processes that we propose account for the abandonment of attempts at weight control and the neglect of weight maintenance as a goal. It contains the following three distinctive elements (none of which, in isolation, is unique to this treatment):

1. *Drawing a distinction between weight loss and weight maintenance.* This distinction is introduced from the outset of treatment and is maintained throughout. It is also inherent in the structure of the treatment, which has two phases. In Phase One (which in the Oxford study involved 17 sessions over 30 weeks) the goal is weight loss. This is followed by a weight maintenance phase during which weight stability is the objective (Phase Two, which in the Oxford study consisted of seven sessions over 14 weeks).

2. *Addressing during the weight loss phase (Phase One) potential obstacles to the acceptance of weight maintenance (i.e., weight stability) as the goal in Phase Two.* This involves:

   a. identifying and moderating unrealistic weight goals;
   b. tackling body image concerns; and
   c. directly addressing patients' primary goals.

Thus in Phase One the therapeutic objective is not just weight loss but also achieving cognitive and behavioral change in other personally salient areas (e.g., appearance, self-confidence, quality of relationships, physical fitness), learning to recognize and value changes that have already been made in treat-

---

[1] A trial evaluating this treatment (the Oxford study) is nearing completion, as described in the Preface.

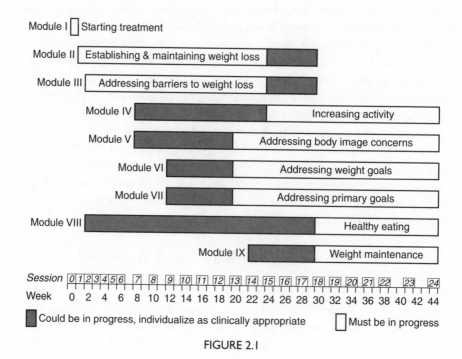

FIGURE 2.1

ment, and learning to accept what cannot be changed (e.g., body proportions). The therapist's goal is that, by the end of Phase One, patients believe that they are able to control their weight to a worthwhile extent and that they accept weight stability rather than weight loss as their subsequent goal.

3. *Helping patients acquire, and then practice, the behavioral skills and cognitive responses needed for effective weight control.* This is the focus of Phase Two. In this phase the therapeutic objective is weight stability and the acquiring of skills to maintain it.

In its style the treatment differs markedly from current behavioral treatments for obesity, as described in Chapter 1. For example, it is administered on an individualized, one-to-one basis, and in therapeutic approach it resembles the cognitive-behavioral treatment for eating disorders.

The remaining chapters of this book specify the strategies and procedures used in the treatment. These are organized into a series of treatment "modules" (see Figure 2.1), which are introduced sequentially and are employed in a flexible way according to the needs of the particular patient.

In the Oxford study, the treatment consisted of 24 sessions (plus an initial assessment session), spread over 44 weeks with the temporal pattern of appointments changing over time. It was our practice to hold appointments at weekly intervals for the first 6 weeks and at 2-week intervals thereafter until week 38, with the final two sessions occurring at 3-week intervals, so that patients had an opportunity to practice managing on their own before treatment ended. With the exception of the assessment session, which took up to 2 hours, each appointment was between 40 and 50 minutes in length.

In our experience the appointment pattern described above suits most patients. However, we are aware that in normal clinical practice the treatment would need to be implemented in a more flexible manner. Some patients would be able to manage with fewer sessions, whereas others would benefit from a longer period of treatment. Thus the pattern of appointments will inevitably deviate from that described in this manual. This is not a cause for concern. On the other hand, it is our view that it is best to avoid breaks in treatment for longer than 3 weeks because momentum tends to get lost. If such a break cannot be avoided, we recommend maintaining therapeutic contact in the interim by use of telephone calls, letters, or E-mail.

Flexibility is also required when implementing the treatment itself. Therapists should personalize the treatment, applying those techniques that are relevant to the individual patient and at a rate that matches their progress. It should be remembered that the various modules do not have to be introduced in the order in which they are numbered here, and most are not expected to be used in isolation. Indeed, aspects of several modules may be discussed during a single session. On the other hand, it is important that all relevant aspects of treatment are covered. Flexibility should not be at the expense of adherence to the overall principles of the treatment.

An Overview of the Treatment

Achieving Weight Loss (Modules I–IV)

As administered in the Oxford study, the weight loss phase of treatment (Phase One) extended over the first 24–30 weeks of treatment. The procedures involved are presented in Modules I–IV (Chapters 3–6). In content these modules are not dissimilar to standard behavioral treatment for obesity (see Wadden & Osei, 2002). Nevertheless we have described them in some detail so that the manual specifies the treatment in its entirety.

In Module I ("Starting Treatment") patients are assessed and the treatment is described with the distinction between weight loss and weight maintenance being introduced and stressed. Detailed self-monitoring of food and fluid intake is introduced and patients are taught how to count calories. Patients are also shown how to plot their weight each week on a graph. This is followed by Module II ("Establishing and Maintaining Weight Loss") in which the emphasis is on helping patients restrict their energy intake to about 1,500 kcal daily. We have found that this level of dietary restriction is sufficient to achieve, on average, a weight loss of 1–2 lb (or 0.5–1 kg)[2] per week. Patients are encouraged to

---

[2] As some clinicians work in pounds and others in kilograms, we have reported both when referring to specific weights. For clarity, we have provided approximate equivalent weights rather than precise conversions (e.g., "2 lb or 1 kg").

devise their own flexible dietary regimen that takes into account their circumstances and food preferences.

Module III ("Addressing Barriers to Weight Loss") runs in parallel with Module II. It focuses on identifying and addressing the various problems that may interfere with patients' adherence to the energy-restricted diet. These include motivational issues, inaccurate monitoring of energy intake, poor food choice (particularly the consumption of a highly restricted range of food or a high-fat diet), excessive alcohol intake, frequent snacking, and eating either as a reward or in response to adverse mood states. "Binge eating" may also be a problem for a subgroup of patients.[3] In our experience, binge eating often resolves without requiring direct attention, although in a small number of cases it is a serious barrier to weight loss and needs to be directly addressed.

A small subgroup of people with obesity meet diagnostic criteria for *binge eating disorder*. This is a new eating disorder diagnosis that technically has provisional status (American Psychiatric Association, 1994). It is primarily characterized by the presence of repeated episodes of binge eating (as defined previously) in the absence of certain other features seen in bulimia nervosa (e.g., repeated self-induced vomiting or laxative misuse; marked and persistent dietary restriction). Binge eating disorder commonly co-occurs with obesity. Nevertheless, its prevalence among patients seeking treatment for obesity is low at about 5–10% (Grilo, 2002). At present there is uncertainty over the best way to help people with binge eating disorder. A variety of psychological treatments show promise (see Dingemans, Bruna, & Van Furth, 2002; Wilfley, 2002), including an adaptation of the cognitive-behavioral treatment for bulimia nervosa (Fairburn et al., 1993; Wilfley et al., 2002), a self-help version of that treatment (Carter and Fairburn, 1998; Fairburn, 1995; Loeb, Wilson, Gilbert, Labouvie, 2000), group interpersonal psychotherapy (Wilfley, MacKenzie, Welch, Ayres, & Weissman, 2000; Wilfley et al., 2002) and, possibly, behavioral weight loss treatment, the latter having the added advantage that it also produces weight loss, at least in the short term. Various pharmacological agents also appear to be effective, although they should probably not be viewed as first-line treatments (Devlin, 2002). In principle, the cognitive-behavioral treatment described in this book should be well suited for patients with both obesity and binge eating disorder (and this is certainly our experience) because, unlike the treatments studied to date, it addresses both the binge eating and the need to lose weight.

Module IV ("Increasing Activity") also forms part of Phase One, although it is primarily concerned with establishing a more active lifestyle in the longer

---

[3] The technical definition of the term *binge* (American Psychiatric Association, 1994) is as follows. "An episode of binge eating is characterized by both of the following: (1) eating, in a discrete period of time (e.g., within any 2-hour period), an amount of food that is definitely larger than most people would eat during a similar period of time and under similar circumstances [and] (2) a sense of lack of control over eating during the episode (e.g., a feeling that one cannot stop eating or control what or how much one is eating)" (p. 731).

term as part of weight maintenance. Thus it is of most relevance to Phase Two. However, it is introduced during Phase One so that there is time for these habits to be consolidated during treatment, as well as to help those patients who want to incorporate lifestyle activity and exercise in their weight loss efforts. The emphasis here is on increasing activity level in general (which necessarily includes decreasing sedentariness) rather than on simply increasing formal exercising.

Addressing Obstacles to the Acceptance of Weight Maintenance (Modules V–VII)

The other three modules that comprise Phase One (Modules V, VI, and VII) are not designed to produce weight loss; rather, they address potential cognitive obstacles to the acceptance of weight maintenance (i.e., weight stability) as a goal in Phase Two. They are employed in a flexible manner both with respect to their timing and the degree of emphasis that is placed on them. Compared with the previous modules, they overlap less in content and style with behavioral treatments for obesity.

Module V ("Addressing Body Image Concerns") is designed to identify and address body image concerns. Concerns about appearance, and in particular a desire to change shape, are a major reason patients want to lose weight (Rosen, 2002). These concerns contribute to their adopting weight goals that are significantly lower than they are likely to achieve (Foster, Wadden, Vogt, & Brewer, 1997). We suggest that unrealistic weight goals, and the concerns they reflect, are major obstacles to patients' recognition and positive acceptance of what they can achieve in treatment.

Module V consists of six partially independent sections and includes a number of established cognitive and behavioral strategies and techniques for addressing these problems (Cash, 1996; Rosen, 1997). Addressing body image concerns, which often needs to be continued over a number of weeks, is always integrated with other aspects of ongoing treatment. It is not introduced in the very early stages of treatment, but once weight loss is well underway (in our experience, at any point between week 8 and week 20; see Figure 2.1).

The focus of Module VI ("Addressing Weight Goals") is on identifying and addressing patients' goals. One of the premises underlying this cognitive-behavioral treatment is that a major obstacle to successful weight maintenance is patients' failure to achieve their weight goals. We have argued that this arises both because they have unrealistic goals for weight loss and because they believe that their other primary goals cannot be achieved without this degree of weight loss. The resulting striving for further weight loss undermines their ability to acquire and use effective weight maintenance strategies (see Cooper & Fairburn, 2001, 2002).

Until recently the belief has been that the appropriate goal weight for a person with obesity is a weight associated with minimum physical morbidity, that is, a BMI in the range 20–25 (the "healthy" range). However, as discussed in Chapter 1, the data indicate that such a goal is unrealistic for most people with obesity (Perri, 2002; Wilson & Brownell, 2002) and that even if they manage to reach this weight, they are unlikely to be able to maintain it for long. By 1-year follow-up, patients typically regain 30–35% of the weight that they have lost (Wadden, Sarwer, & Berkowitz, 1999) and, for the majority of patients, weight regain continues thereafter until most or all of the lost weight has been regained.

The aim of Module VI is to help patients adopt and accept a more appropriate weight goal, and to recognize that many of their primary goals can be achieved independently of weight loss. The timing of the introduction of this module varies according to the progress of the individual patient and the extent to which unrealistic weight goals become an issue in treatment. It has been our practice to introduce it some time between weeks 12 and 20 (see Figure 2.1).

The patient's primary goals are addressed in Module VII ("Addressing Primary Goals"). Primary goals are objectives that patients hope to achieve as a result of weight loss. They include changing appearance, improving self-confidence, enhancing interpersonal functioning, and increasing fitness. The aim of Module VII is to help patients directly address these goals. We suggest that this is an essential element in treatment as it is likely to result in greater satisfaction with what has been accomplished (irrespective of whether patients' initial weight loss goal has been reached) and, therefore, better acceptance of weight maintenance as an objective in Phase Two. Although primary goals are discussed in outline as part of the initial assessment process, they are not formally addressed until weight loss is well underway. Thus this module is usually introduced in the course of discussing weight goals (in our experience between weeks 12 and 20), and runs concurrently with it (see Figure 2.1).

In Module VIII ("Healthy Eating") the focus is on healthy eating in the long term, although selected elements from this module may be introduced during the weight loss phase if they are needed to promote weight loss. This module follows standard contemporary nutritional guidelines (U.S. Department of Agriculture, 1995). The key recommendations are to eat less fat, and to consume plenty of fruit and vegetables, as well as foods from the bread, cereal, rice, and pasta group.

Weight Maintenance (Module IX)

The most distinctive feature of this cognitive-behavioral treatment is the priority it gives to long-term weight maintenance. This topic is raised at the beginning of treatment when it is explained that the treatment has both a weight loss phase and a weight maintenance phase, and it is addressed during weight loss when potential cognitive barriers to long-term weight maintenance are tackled (Modules V–VII). During Phase Two weight maintenance is the focus of treatment, with patients being strongly discouraged from attempting to lose further weight, whatever their weight loss has been up to this point.

The introduction of Module IX ("Weight Maintenance") coincides with entering Phase Two and is unique to it. The point at which the module is entered varies according to individual need. Our practice is always to enter this module between weeks 24 and 30, thereby allowing a minimum of 14 weeks before the end of treatment for the acquisition and practice of weight maintenance skills.

In preparation for weight maintenance, the differences between losing weight and maintaining a stable weight are highlighted. There are three major differences: First, weight maintenance is less reinforcing than weight loss, in part because there is less encouragement from others; second, the process of weight maintenance is indefinite, rather than time limited; and third, it may involve accepting a weight and shape that was previously regarded as unacceptable (Wadden, 1995). Difficulties commonly encountered with long-term weight control are also discussed.

An essential first step in weight maintenance is to define a specific target weight range and establish a weight monitoring system that provides patients with the information needed to keep their weight within this target range. Patients are helped to distinguish significant changes in their weight from trivial fluctuations and encouraged to take corrective action when necessary.

To rehearse the strategies needed to respond to weight change, patients are presented with possible future scenarios involving either changes in weight or obstacles to weight monitoring. Adopting this future-oriented perspective, patients are also encouraged to think ahead about a number of difficult issues that could arise after treatment has ended. Patients are asked to consider the relative merits of actively keeping their weight within the agreed range by thinking and planning ahead, as opposed to allowing their weight to change and then having to react by making the necessary adjustments. They are also asked to identify whether any aspect of their behavior or attitudes, such as a tendency to overeat in response to stress or to consume high-fat snacks, might put them at particular risk of weight regain.

Drawing up a personal weight maintenance plan is another aspect of planning for the future. Patients are informed of the value of having such a plan, in particular that it provides a useful reminder of what they have learned about weight maintenance as well as being a guide about what to do in the future. The maintenance plan is developed collaboratively and always has a section on weight maintenance and one on dealing with setbacks.

The Remainder of the Book

The remainder of this book describes the new treatment in detail. As noted in the preface, we have kept references to the clinical and research literature to a minimum so as to present the material in a way that makes the manual easy to use. For the convenience of readers, where we have included references, we have tried as far as possible to confine them to one text, *Eating Disorders and Obesity: A Comprehensive Handbook* (Fairburn & Brownell, 2002), because this book contains many relevant summary chapters written by experts in the field. In addition, each chapter has guidelines for further reading. We hope that we have thus provided readers with good sources of further information without their having to pursue large numbers of individual references.

CHAPTER 3

Module I: Starting Treatment

Module I	Starting treatment	

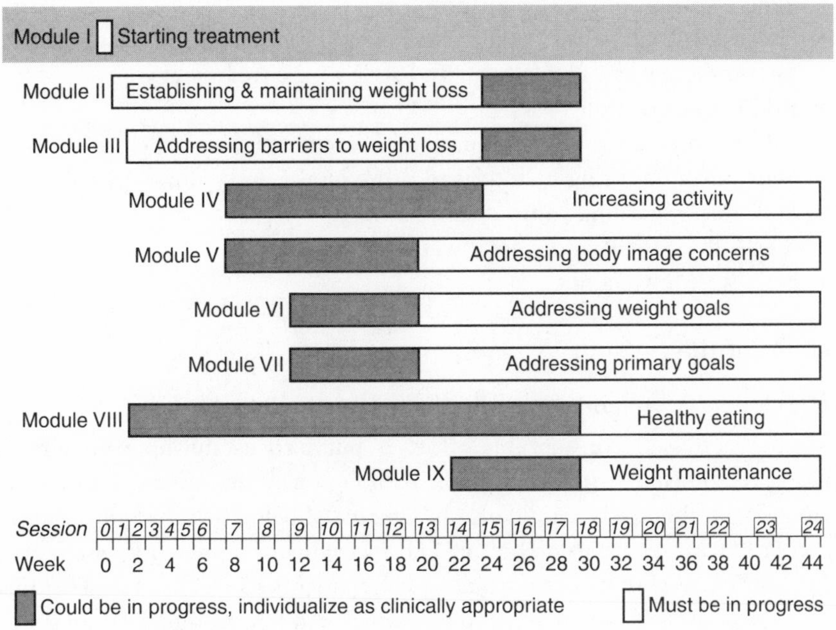

FIGURE 3.1

In the Oxford study, we began treatment with two preparatory sessions (sessions 0 and 1) before weight loss is initiated (see Figure 3.1). These two sessions have the following goals:

1. To establish an effective working relationship.
2. To orient the patient to the treatment.
3. To enhance motivation.
4. To assess the weight problem.
5. To establish the monitoring of eating habits and energy intake.
6. To establish weekly weighing.

Once these goals have been achieved to a reasonably satisfactory extent, the patient embarks upon losing weight.

Session 0: Assessment and Orientation

This session may take up to 2 hours to allow time for the initial history taking. Its structure differs from the standard format used in future sessions. As the session is long, it may be appropriate to have a short break at some point (e.g., before the setting of homework assignments).

Overview of the Session

- Develop a collaborative working relationship.
- Take a history of the weight problem.
- Describe in outline the cognitive-behavioral perspective on weight control.
- Orient the patient to the form and style of the treatment.
- Address motivation.
- Address premature discontinuation of treatment.
- Start self-monitoring of food and drink intake and calorie counting.
- Forewarn regarding calorie restriction.
- Weigh the patient and start a weight graph.
- Start weekly weighing.

Content of the Session

Developing a Collaborative Therapist–Patient Relationship

From the outset, considerable effort is put into establishing an effective working relationship with the patient. Although genuine interest and concern are important, therapists should also be capable of being firm and authoritative, particularly with regard to the setting and reviewing of homework assignments.

In this first session it is important to help patients to feel at ease. Therapists will need to use their judgment as to how much can be accomplished. In general it is important to allow time to answer patients' questions and not to over-whelm them with questions, handouts, and homework assignments.

Assessing the History and Character of the Weight Problem

The therapist should ask the patient for a brief description of the weight problem and how it is affecting his or her life. Table 3.1 lists topics that it is helpful to cover. The major focus of the questioning should be on the patient's weight history, weight loss attempts, weight goals, and attitudes to shape and weight. It is not expected that everything of interest or relevance will emerge in this one session.

The history taking will enable the therapist to:

- ensure that this treatment is suitable, in particular to exclude those who should be treated for an eating disorder other than binge eating disorder (see page 10);
- begin to forge an effective therapist–patient relationship;
- gauge the nature and severity of the weight problem;

- begin to identify the patient's treatment goals (i.e., weight and shape-related goals and "primary" goals, for example, to have more self-respect, to find a partner, to change jobs, etc.); and
- begin to relate the cognitive-behavioral model of weight control to the particular patient's difficulties controlling his or her weight (i.e., the creation of a personalized formulation).[1]

A 63-year-old patient described having struggled to control her weight since her childhood. She also described long-standing insecurity about her self-worth. About 3 years earlier, she had sought psychotherapy to help her explore and address her insecurities. This had been a great success. When asked why she wanted to lose weight she answered that there were two reasons: first, to improve her health (she had hypertension) and, second, to improve her appearance (especially her bust size). On reflection, she then said that neither was the primary reason. Instead, the reason she wanted to lose weight was to gain self-respect. She thought that her weight problem represented the "last frontier," the only remaining expression of her difficulties accepting herself as being of value. For this patient, controlling her eating and weight were of great personal significance.

Orienting the Patient to the Treatment

Rationale for the Treatment. The therapist should explain that there are two aspects to the treatment of being overweight[2]—losing weight and then maintaining the weight that has been lost. The former (losing weight) is comparatively straightforward for many people, whereas the latter (maintaining the weight lost) is much more difficult. In other words, the key issue in long-term weight control is generally maintaining a new weight after having lost weight rather than weight loss per se. It is for this reason that this treatment makes a distinction between weight loss and weight maintenance, and accordingly there is a weight loss phase in treatment followed by a weight maintenance phase. Patients should be told that toward the end of treatment they will be asked to stop trying to lose weight, so that they have sufficient time in treatment to learn to keep their weight stable. This emphasis on weight maintenance distinguishes the treatment from other approaches (which pay relatively little attention to weight maintenance).

---

[1] At this stage the personalized formulation is less detailed and specific than is usual in cognitive-behavioral treatments. This is because the priority at this point is to initiate weight loss. A more complete formulation is presented and discussed when weight goals are considered (see Chapter 8).

[2] Many patients find the term *obesity* distressing or distasteful, and so it is generally better to avoid the term and use the word *overweight* instead.

TABLE 3.1

Assessment Checklist

1. History of weight problem

- Development of the weight problem
  - How the problem began
  - When the problem began (age and year)
  - What was happening at the time
- Subsequent course
  - Subsequent evolution of the problem (i.e., history until the present)
  - Pattern of weight change (e.g., steady unrelenting increase, fluctuations up and down, periods of weight stability)
  - Highest and lowest weight (since patient reached present height)
- Prior attempts to lose weight and their outcome
  - General account of the nature and duration of these attempts
  - Effect on weight (amount lost, weight attained, and degree of satisfaction)
  - Success at weight maintenance (duration of maintenance)
  - Weight regain (triggers, rapidity of regain)

2. Current state

- Eating habits (ask about a typical day)
  - Eating pattern (e.g., meals and snacks eaten, eating outside meals, variability from day to day, weekdays vs. weekends)
  - Amounts eaten (including idea of portion sizes)
  - Food choice
  - Episodes of loss of control over eating and amounts eaten
  - Nature of current attempts to restrict eating
  - Other problems with eating (e.g., self-induced vomiting, misuse of laxatives or diuretics)
- Physical activity
  - Nature and frequency of current physical activity, including both lifestyle activity (i.e., occupational and recreational activity) and formal exercising (e.g., swimming, exercise classes)
  - Attitude toward physical activity and exercise
- Reasons for wanting to lose weight
  - To change appearance (e.g., to feel more attractive, to change clothes size, to be more attractive to others)
  - To achieve another personal objective (e.g., relating to work, personal relationships, sporting activities, or to improve self-respect)
  - To improve a health problem or reduce the risk of illness
  - Other reasons (e.g., to reduce physical discomfort or to escape the discrimination associated with being overweight)
- Attitude toward appearance
  - Views on overall shape and body parts
  - Importance of shape and weight in personal self-evaluation
- Weight and weight goals (see Chapter 8 for definitions)
  - Current weight
  - Ideal (or "dream") weight
  - True goal weight ("desired weight")
  - How patients think their life would change if they reached their desired weight
  - What a realistic weight goal would be, all things considered
  - What the minimum acceptable weight loss would be
- Physical health
  - Current medical problems (including psychiatric problems)
  - Current treatment (medication, other treatments)
  - Medical history (including psychiatric history)

continued

TABLE 3.1

——————

(continued)

- Smoking and drinking
  - Current smoking and drinking habits (amount, pattern)
- Relationship between smoking and weight problem

3. Other information that may have a bearing on treatment

- Social circumstances
  - Occupation and working hours
  - Where the patient lives and ease of transport (to sessions)
  - Marital status and attitude of spouse (or significant other) toward treatment
  - Living arrangements (i.e., who is at home)
  - Children
  - Interests
- Foreseeable barriers to weight loss
  - Personal (e.g., poor motivation, hopelessness, low mood)
  - External (e.g., difficulties at home, stress at work, food-related occupation)
- Family history of obesity and eating problems
  - Weight and eating problems in first degree relatives

4. Anything else that the patient sees as important

To bolster the rationale for the treatment, the therapist should refer to any prior difficulties that the patient has experienced maintaining his or her weight following weight loss. The therapist should explain how this form of treatment is designed to address such difficulties. In the first phase of treatment, although the main emphasis is on weight loss, there is also a focus on establishing the types of habits and attitudes that are likely to help subsequent weight maintenance. Later on, the focus is almost exclusively weight maintenance. The patient will be helped to acquire weight maintenance skills and any difficulty applying these skills will be addressed. It is helpful for the therapist to give examples of factors that may lead to weight regain, drawing on the patient's experience in the past. It should be made clear that such factors are generally both behavioral (i.e., not doing the right things) and cognitive (e.g., having unrealistic goals and expectations, a poor body image, or reacting inappropriately to signs of weight gain) in nature.[3] Patients should be told that the aim is to make permanent changes in their thinking about weight control as well as in their eating and activity so that they will be able to maintain their new weight in the long term.

An account was obtained of a patient's previous attempts to maintain her new weight following weight loss. She reported that she had not previously thought about long-term weight maintenance, and it had never been emphasized by any of the treatments that she had followed.

---

[3] Therapists should avoid using technical terms (such as *behavioral, cognitive, cognitive-behavioral,* etc.) and should instead use concrete examples the patient is likely to relate to.

> In the past she had simply stopped dieting. She would then discover that she was gaining weight and, if anything, she thought that this led her to overeat rather than restart dieting.
>
> The therapist commented that difficulties of this type are extremely common and that they would be explicitly addressed in treatment. Indeed, the main emphasis of the latter half of treatment would be on weight maintenance as the goal was enduring weight change rather than weight loss followed by weight regain.

Treatment Structure.   Patients should be informed of the number of sessions available to them, and the frequency of appointments. (For example, as described in Chapter 2, it has been our practice to offer an assessment followed by 24 sessions over 44 weeks. The first six sessions have been weekly, and the remainder have been biweekly except for the last two sessions, which have been 3 weeks apart.) If patients are unable to commit themselves to attending appointments regularly over the planned time period, it may be unwise to begin treatment. In order for treatment to succeed, it needs to be a major priority in the patient's life. The therapist should ask the patient about any periods of travel that might disrupt treatment. If a trip is coming up, it might be better to postpone the start of treatment until after the patient has returned.

Patients should also be informed of the length of appointments. (In our case this is 40–50 minutes.) Our practice has been to inform patients that sessions will always end on time, and that it is up to the patient and therapist to ensure that they begin on time. This is also a good time to ask patients how they would like to be addressed (first name or surname) and to say how the therapist would like to be addressed.

Style of the Treatment.   The therapist should emphasize that the treatment is collaborative in nature with the patient being expected to play an active role in determining the content of the sessions and the nature of homework assignments. It should be stressed that treatment requires commitment and a change in lifestyle. Half-hearted attempts at treatment tend to fail. Regular and individualized homework assignments will be agreed upon at the end of each treatment session, and it is expected that patients will do their utmost to complete them. The more effort that is put into treatment, the greater the rewards are likely to be. The therapist will provide information, advice, and encouragement, but it is up to the patient to make the most of this opportunity to change.[4]

---

[4] The use of E-mail as an adjunct or alternative to face-to-face psychological treatment is attracting interest (Shafran, 2002; Yager, 2001). It is certainly a way of communicating about practical arrangements (e.g., appointment times), and it can be used to maintain momentum between sessions, but there can also be complications. For example, patients may E-mail their therapist when facing a personal crisis, hoping for an immediate response. We urge therapists to be cautious in this regard and recommend that the ground rules for using E-mail are made absolutely clear at the outset when exchanging E-mail addresses.

TABLE 3.2
───────
An Example List of Pros and Cons

Pros	Cons
Lose some weight	Too much effort
Look better	Too busy
Be healthier	Will complicate social situations

Likely Outcome.   Patients should be told that, during the weight loss phase, they can expect to achieve a weight loss of about 1–2 lb (0.5–1 kg) a week, although there is considerable variation from person to person and from week to week. People also vary in how long they can keep this up. Once patients have lost weight, the key question is whether they can avoid weight regain in the future. Other treatments generally fail in this regard. This treatment is designed to minimize the risk of weight regain. However, for the meantime the patient should focus his or her efforts on getting going with treatment since our experience suggests that those who work hard from the beginning do best.

Addressing Motivation

On being presented with all this information, there is a risk that patients will feel overwhelmed. It is therefore important to ask them for their views on the prospect of treatment and in particular the level of commitment required. If the therapist senses some degree of ambivalence, then the patient's level of motivation definitely needs to be addressed. On the other hand, if it is clear that the patient is motivated, then the therapist can move straight on to the next topic— while bearing in mind that motivation is not fixed. Even if it is not a problem at this point, it may become one later on.

If motivation appears to be an issue, then it should be actively discussed, and the patient's concerns and reservations explored. To address motivation, the therapist should raise the subject directly and help the patient list all the pros and cons of treatment, from his or her perspective. The pros and cons can be written down in a simple table, such as the one shown in Table 3.2.

It is important to explore each of the listed items, starting with the "cons." Full details of each con should be obtained from the patient. Then the same should be done with the "pros," with the therapist taking the lead. The therapist should make sure that both short-term and long-term time frames are adopted. In general patients are able to see that the cons are mainly immediate, whereas the benefits are likely to be both short term (e.g., weight loss, looking better) and long term (e.g., maintenance of the new lower weight rather than oscillating up and down; improved health; enhanced appearance and self-esteem).

When examining the pros and cons, the therapist should be careful to adopt an exploratory and even-handed style. The therapist should not be prescriptive, as this might interfere with rapport and create defensiveness, and the process should not be rushed.

In some cases the problem with motivation stems from practical difficulties attending treatment. Such difficulties should be addressed using a problem-solving approach (see Chapter 4, section on developing problem-solving skills).

Patients whose motivation remains in doubt should be asked to think further about the matter over the next week (and elaborate the pros and cons list, taking care to include a long-term perspective), and they should be encouraged to discuss the issue with family members and relevant others. In our experience it is best to delay starting treatment until patients have fully made up their minds one way or other. For these patients, the session should end at this point.

Addressing Premature Discontinuation of Treatment

Related to motivation is the topic of prematurely discontinuing treatment. This subject needs to be raised as a matter of routine with the hope that doing so will minimize unwarranted attrition later on.

If the patient thinks he or she might be tempted to give up, possible reasons for this should be discussed. "Not doing well enough" may reflect unrealistic standards rather than poor performance; weight regained can often be rapidly "re-lost," so long as prompt action is taken; and feeling overwhelmed with other life commitments calls for a thorough examination of one's priorities, adopting a long-term as well as short-term perspective, rather than the abandonment of treatment. The therapist should stress the need for the patient to be open about any urges to drop out.

Starting Self-Monitoring of Food and Drink Intake

It should be explained to the patient that there are two cornerstones to this type of treatment. One is the accurate monitoring of energy intake (i.e., writing down all food and drink consumed) and the other is regular weighing.

Writing down everything that is consumed is valuable for many reasons:

- It helps patients change.
- It increases patients' awareness of their behavior.
- It enhances control over eating.
- It identifies which behaviors and patterns of thinking need to be tackled.
- It helps the therapist and patient examine the patient's behavior, thinking, and progress, and the circumstances under which problems arise.
- It helps patients see what positive changes they are making.
- It allows patients to identify their main sources of calories. This will be of great help in planning how they can lose weight and then keep their weight stable in the long term.

The therapist must stress that recording what is eaten is fundamental to treatment. Without good recording, treatment is likely to fail. Research shows that the more effort people put in to treatment, the more they will get out of it.

TABLE 3.3
_____

Instructions for Self-Monitoring

RECORDING YOUR EATING

The importance of recording cannot be stressed too much. It is vital if treatment is to succeed. Recording will help you identify exactly which aspects of your behavior you need to change, *and it will help you make these changes.*

At this stage you need to record everything that you eat and drink. A simple description will do. To do this, you will need to carry your records with you. The following instructions are to help you complete the records.

- Column 1 is for noting the exact time of day you ate or drank the items concerned. You should write things down as soon as possible afterward.
- Column 2 is for giving a simple description of what was eaten and drunk. You should record absolutely everything consumed. Please identify meals with brackets.
- Column 3 is for noting where you were at the time. If at home, please note the room.
- An asterisk should be placed in column 4 beside anything you ate or drank that you viewed as excessive. This should be your view not other people's.
- Column 5 is for noting calories.
- Column 6 is for noting other points of relevance (e.g., your thoughts or feelings, the circumstances, or context in which the eating occurred). You should also note your weight in this column each time that you weigh yourself.

Please remember to bring your records to each treatment session.

_____

In particular, people who self-monitor carefully and accurately are likely to lose significantly more weight than those who do not (Boutelle & Kirschenbaum, 1998).

The patient should then be given a copy of the handout "Recording Your Eating" (see Table 3.3; Handout A[5]) together with copies of the two example food diaries (see Figures 3.2 and 3.3; Handouts B and C). The therapist should use these forms to explain how the food diaries should be completed, while giving the patient an opportunity to ask questions. It is important to stress that the records should be completed "prospectively" (i.e., soon after eating, rather than some hours later) because this type of recording is most accurate and best helps people examine and change their behavior and ways of thinking.

The patient should also be given a supply of blank recording forms to use (Handout D). (Alternatively, patients can be asked to photocopy the forms themselves.) Finally the patient should be asked to begin recording the following day.

Potential difficulties with recording should be discussed, with the patient being invited to foresee any problems that are likely to arise. Some patients may express concern that recording will make them preoccupied with eating and that this will be counterproductive. Therapists should acknowledge that a tem-

_____

[5] The patient handouts are to be found in Appendix I.

DAY Wednesday   DATE 7th October

Time	Food and Drink Consumed	Place	*	Calories	Comments
8.45 am.	2 slices brown bread	kitchen	*	160	Did not really want it
	14g butter		*	102	
	14g peanut butter		*	87	Eating without thinking.
	water			0	
8.55					Weight 103kg Too heavy.
10.50	Diet coke	work			
12.50	Chocolate from vending machine	work	*	255	Calories on pack. I had planned to go to canteen, but 4 people I knew were there and I didn't want them to see me eat.
1p.m.	prawn mayonnaise sandwich (low fat)	In town		283	Calories on pack
	diet coke			0	
	chocolate bar		*	255	Did not want it, do not know why I ate it.
15.00	Diet coke	work		0	
18.05	1 gin and tonic	pub		85	Out with colleagues. Did not enjoy it – I was thinking about my food problems
19.40	Half a loaf of bread (i.e. 400g)	dining room	*	880	I estimated calories as I did not weigh it. I feel awful. I cannot believe I've done this again.
	butter		*	510	
	peanut butter		*	435	
	4 glasses red wine		*	340	
		TOTAL		3392	I'm going to bed.

FIGURE 3.2   Example food diary

DAY Sunday   DATE 15th August

Time	Food and Drink Consumed	Place	*	Calories	Comments
10 a.m.	2 slices toast	front room		158	
	cream cheese (light)			25	
	black coffee			0	
11.40 am	10 Pringles	front room		110	Saw them and could not resist!
Noon	nectarine	kitchen		80	Think I was just bored.
1.40	2 slices toast	front room		158	
	cream cheese (light)			25	
	diet coke			0	
6.30	chicken (9oz)	front room		306	Very satisfying Meal
	roast potatoes (4oz)			172	
	carrots (8oz)			80	
	cauliflower (9oz)			90	
7.20	large orange (13oz)	kitchen		91	
9pm	medium banana	friend's house		114	I couldn't weigh this, so calories are an estimate.
9.40	glass of wine (medium, white)	friend's house		95	
		TOTAL		1504	I'm pleased with today

FIGURE 3.3   Example food diary

porary increase in preoccupation may occur, but this soon wanes. Patients should be encouraged to keep their monitoring records private as they will be asked to record relevant thoughts and feelings later on, and these are likely to be quite personal. They should carry their records with them at all times and should bring them to each session. It should also be explained that the therapist will be keeping the records.[6]

Some patients are reluctant to monitor their food intake, especially if they are ashamed about the way that they eat. The therapist should anticipate this response by assuring patients that there is no need to be ashamed of their behavior, and by telling them that recording what actually happens is an essential first step in addressing their problems and overcoming them.

Some patients may believe that recording will be hard work or not sufficiently worthwhile to justify the effort. Some say that they have recorded in the past and did not find it helpful. The reply should be that it is most unlikely that they have monitored in the way that is being proposed or that they have used the information in the way it will be used in this treatment. It should again be stressed that self-monitoring is central to the treatment and it is essential if their weight problem is to be tackled. In fact, patients are often surprised at how helpful recording is, and some are reluctant to give it up at the end of treatment.

One patient described herself as being "out of control" and explained that she frequently ate snacks in order to cope with feelings of agitation or anxiety. After her first week of recording, she was very positive about the diary keeping. She reported that she felt much more "in control," and had eaten fewer snacks as a result.

Another patient was initially slightly dubious about the process of recording on the grounds that she was a seasoned dieter and felt she was well aware of the calorie values of the food she ate. She returned after the first week feeling that she had really learned something valuable. She had first written down what she estimated her food intake to be on an average day and calculated the calorie content for this. The total had come to approximately 1,200 calories. She had then recorded as the therapist had asked her, noting every single item of food and drink, and again assessed the calorie content. The total was considerably higher than 1,200. The patient recognized that when assessing her "average" day (i.e., what she imagined she was generally eating) she had not taken account of the many "extras" she consumed during the course of the day.

---

[6] It is our practice to keep the patient's self-monitoring records so that they are available for reference during future treatment sessions should this seem useful. For instance, referring back to earlier records can help highlight the patient's progress. Or, if the patient's daily calorie intake has increased, it can be helpful to refer to earlier records to remind him or her of lower-calorie food choices he or she was making earlier.

Starting Counting Calories

The therapist should provide the patient with detailed guidelines for counting his or her calorie intake. This part of the session must not be hurried. The patient should be given a "user-friendly" calorie guide, and shown how to use it.[7] Patients will definitely need a kitchen food-weighing scale and if they do not have one, then they should be asked to buy one as soon as possible. At this point it is also worth informing patients that most people significantly underestimate their food intake. They should therefore be on the alert for this possibility and counter it by adjusting their estimate upward whenever they are uncertain about how much they have eaten.

Occasionally therapists may decide to delay calorie counting until the next treatment session. This is advisable if there is insufficient time left to explain calorie counting, or if it seems likely that the patient will find calorie counting very difficult. In such instances the patient should be asked (as homework) to record everything he or she eats and drinks, without working out the calorie content. However, in the vast majority of cases it is appropriate to introduce calorie counting during this initial session.

Preparing the Patient for Calorie Restriction

The therapist should explain that there is no need for the patient to change his or her eating this week. Instead, he or she should focus on becoming expert at monitoring and calorie counting, as that is enough to have to concentrate on this week. However, the patient should be informed that at the next session he or she will be asked to start reducing calorie intake to about 1,500 calories daily. (If the patient has a baseline intake substantially higher than this, a higher initial calorie goal may be chosen; see session 1.) In the meantime he or she should eat as usual while developing ideas about how best to adapt to meeting this lower calorie goal. These ideas will then be reviewed with the therapist at the next session.

Weighing the Patient and Starting a Weight Graph

As will become clear, a central feature of this treatment is that patients should know their weight and learn how to interpret individual readings on the scale. Usually sessions start with patients being weighed, but on this occasion patients should be weighed toward the end of the session. They should be told their weight, and the therapist should record it on a graph. (This graph should have the date or week of treatment along the horizontal axis, and the patient's weight along the vertical one.)

---

[7] The characteristics of a good calorie guide are that it should be reasonably comprehensive in the foods listed; it should be arranged so that it is easy to find particular foods within it (e.g., alphabetical, with sensible groupings); and calories should be given by weight and, when servings are always of a similar size, per serving (e.g., one cookie of a particular variety, or for an average apple). It is best if it does not include unnecessary detail (e.g., information on macronutrient composition).

Starting Weekly Weighing

Therapists should explain that although patients will be weighed at each session, they should also weigh themselves at home at weekly intervals. This is the second cornerstone of treatment. Weekly weighing is designed to help patients monitor the changes in their weight when losing weight but, more importantly, it is central to the stabilization of weight as part of weight maintenance during Phase Two (see Chapter 11).

Patients should be told that weekly weighing is recommended (on a specific weekday morning of their choice) because this frequency of weighing provides the right amount of information to detect changes in their weight over time. Less frequent weighing provides insufficient feedback for this stage in treatment, whereas weighing more often than this can lead to patients becoming preoccupied with trivial day-to-day weight fluctuations, which in turn can interfere with dietary compliance. For example, patients may feel disheartened by days on which there is apparent weight gain or no weight loss, although such days are not uncommon even among those who are complying with the energy restriction. Many factors affect body weight in the short term (e.g., the patient's state of hydration and point in the menstrual cycle), and these can disguise or exaggerate apparent progress.

Patients should be forewarned that it is impossible to interpret individual weight readings, as for a variety of reasons, body weight fluctuates significantly from day to day and within the day, and one cannot therefore know whether any single reading is a peak, a trough, or somewhere in between. One needs to look at trends over longer periods of time, three or four readings at weekly intervals being the minimum.

If patients do not have a scale, they should be told that they will need to buy one. Perfectly adequate scales can be bought reasonably cheaply.

It is not unusual for there to be a discrepancy between the weight recorded on the therapist's and patient's scales. This is not a problem so long as the size of the discrepancy remains constant. If it does not, patients should be asked to buy a new, more accurate scale.

Each time they weigh themselves, patients should note their weight on the right-hand column of the day's monitoring record. They should also plot it on a graph. The therapist should teach them how to do this. It involves writing either the date or week of treatment on the horizontal axis each time that they plot their weight.[8]

---

[8] The therapist and patient should together decide whether it would be better to plot the patient's actual weight (as shown on the scale) or the change in the patient's weight since the last reading. If the patient intends to leave the graph where it might be seen by others, the latter may be preferable. Plotting weight change is also experienced by many patients as more encouraging.

Ending the Session

Therapists should do their utmost to ensure that this session and all subsequent sessions end on a positive note. Patients should leave feeling encouraged, optimistic, and clear about what they are to do. They should also have had an opportunity to ask questions.

The therapist should provide a brief summary of the session, so that the patient has a clear understanding of the topics covered. It is generally not realistic to expect the patient to be able to summarize the session at this stage, but this may be appropriate as treatment progresses. The patient should be reminded that this session was exceptionally long and that future sessions will last no longer than 50 minutes. The therapist should also explain that future sessions will have a fairly standard format (as in the cognitive-behavioral treatment of bulimia nervosa [Wilson et al., 1997]; see Chapter 4). Finally, the therapist should ensure that the patient is absolutely clear about the homework that has been agreed upon. Generally this will involve the following:

1. Monitoring of food and drink intake, including calorie counting
2. Weekly weighing

Next Appointment

Our practice is to see the patient again in 4–7 days.

Session 1

Overview of the Session

- Weigh the patient and record the patient's weight on the weight graph.
- Check whether the patient has weighed her- or himself at home.
- Jointly review the self-monitoring records.
- Set agenda for session collaboratively.
- Work through agenda topics.
- Agree on new homework assignments.
- Summarize the session.

In session 1, most of the time should be devoted to a thorough review of the patient's monitoring records (about 30 minutes). As always, it is important to ask the patient what she or he would like to put on the agenda. The therapist's main agenda items this session should be to identify and address concerns about treatment; to provide a brief account of the health risks associated with obesity; and to advise the patient to start restricting calorie intake to an average of 1,500 calories daily (unless a higher calorie goal is appropriate). There should be a brief discussion as to how this can be achieved. As always, it is important not to overwhelm the patient. The amount of material covered must be adjusted to suit the particular patient.

At the same time, therapists should do their best to build up their relationship with the patient. They should be encouraging and should highlight and praise everything that the patient has achieved. Self-monitoring and calorie counting should receive particular attention.

Patients whose motivation was in doubt in the initial session should have the first part of this session devoted to a further review of the pros and cons of change. Then, assuming that they wish to continue with treatment, they should be given the homework assignments associated with that session (i.e., self-monitoring, calorie counting, and weekly weighing). In other words they should continue where they finished off in the previous session, and they should progress on to session 1 material 1 week later than the majority of patients.

If motivation still appears to be an issue, it should be the subject of the entire session. There is no point embarking on treatment if the patient is a reluctant participant.

Content of the Session

Weighing the Patient

The patient should be weighed at the beginning of the session under the same conditions as before. The therapist should enter the weight onto the weight graph (while the patient watches). This graph may be annotated with explanatory notes (e.g., vacation, birthday) if relevant.

In this session little time should be devoted to the subject of weight. No weight change is to be expected, although some loss is not uncommon through the effects that self-monitoring and calorie counting have on eating. If there is weight loss, the therapist should respond positively. If the patient's weight is unchanged or has increased, the therapist should also be encouraging noting that starting to reduce calorie intake is on the agenda for this session.

Weighing at Home

Before addressing the patient's monitoring, this is a natural point to raise the issue of weighing at home. The regular self-monitoring of weight is important and needs to be established early on. Weekly weighing is recommended (see session 0 for the reasons for this) with patients recording their weight on their personal weight graph. Patients should be reminded not to draw inferences about their weight on the basis of less than four consecutive weekly readings (i.e., they should only draw conclusions on the basis of trends over time rather than from isolated readings).

Patients who are weighing themselves more often than once a week need to be advised that this is not a good idea. They may find it difficult to restrict weighing themselves to once a week, because they fear that they will gain inordinate amounts of weight between each weighing. This fear can be put to the test. Such patients may need to keep their scales out of sight to help them resist weighing themselves too often. However, at this stage in treatment too frequent weighing need not be a major source of concern. Therapists should explain that they will be returning to the subject of weighing later on in treatment (see Chapter 7).

Some patients actively avoid weighing themselves. This is indicative of extreme concern about weight. It is much more problematic for treatment than too frequent weighing as knowledge of weight is central to the treatment process. It is needed for patients to learn the relationship between their energy intake and their weight; and it is required when addressing the relationship between shape and weight and when examining patients' weight goals (see Chapter 8). The need for patients to know their weight and monitor it must be stressed by the therapist. It is a prerequisite for treatment. Although it may be tempting for therapists to acquiesce to certain patients' strong wish not to know their weight (perhaps thinking that the issue can be tackled later), this temptation should be resisted. Treatment cannot continue without patients monitoring their weight. Patients should be forewarned that on starting to weigh themselves they may well experience an increase in the intensity of their concerns about their weight and perhaps even an urge to weigh themselves more often than once a week, but that this is likely to be short-lived.

Reviewing the Monitoring Records

After the introduction of self-monitoring in the assessment session, each subsequent appointment should open with a review of the monitoring records that have been completed since the last session. The records should be discussed in great detail in the first few sessions (as described in Fairburn et al., 1993). The purpose is twofold. One goal is to obtain an accurate picture of the patient's eating habits; and the second is to encourage and reinforce the patient's compliance with this seminal homework assignment. Systematic self-monitoring is central to the success of this treatment for the reasons discussed earlier, and the quality of a patient's monitoring is related in a large part to the amount of attention that the therapist pays to it. Establishing detailed and accurate self-monitoring is the foundation for compliance with the remainder of the treatment.

As noted in session 0, some patients may be embarrassed about their eating and might therefore have failed to record accurately. If the recording of energy intake underestimates the amount being consumed, the therapist and patient will get a misleading impression of his or her behavioral compliance and the relationship between energy intake and weight loss. Overestimation of energy intake also sometimes occurs, and it can lead patients to exercise excessive calorie restriction. The detailed review of the monitoring records helps identify likely inaccuracies and should lead to more accurate recording in the future.

Therapists should therefore be painstaking when reviewing the first set of records. They should check when food items were written down (i.e., how long after they were consumed), the accuracy of the description, and whether there are any omissions. This should not be done in a critical or judgmental manner.

The therapist should remind the patient of the importance of writing down what they ate immediately after they have eaten it, rather than in retrospect. Only in this way will the full benefits of monitoring be obtained—a major purpose of monitoring is to help patients keep track of what they are doing as they go along. Any difficulties with monitoring should be explored and solutions sought. Accurate monitoring should be strongly praised.

It is most effective for the patient to take the lead in guiding the therapist through each day's record. The therapist should facilitate this process by asking questions where points are unclear. This detailed review is not only informative in its own right, but it also conveys the importance of accurate calorie counting.

When reviewing the monitoring records, the therapist should have the following general questions in mind:

1. *Is the patient recording everything?* Therapists should regularly ask patients this specific question. All suspected inaccuracies should be explored. There may be straightforward errors (e.g., simply forgetting to record an episode of eating), or there may be purposeful minimization or omission. Episodes of excessive eating (particularly binge eating) are especially likely to be omitted. The accurate monitoring of all episodes of eating and drinking is needed not only for the calculation of energy intake but also to identify behavioral obstacles to compliance such as binge eating, picking, and stress-related eating.

2. *Is the patient accurately assessing portion sizes?* This is essential for the calculation of energy intake. It is a laborious process, and it requires weighing food. For understandable reasons most patients gradually abandon such weighing as the weeks pass. In some cases this results in a gradual increase in portion size that goes undetected and can make a significant contribution to the inevitable decline in the rate of weight loss over time. Therapists should therefore regularly ask patients how they are calculating their portion sizes, and potential sources of error should be explored and addressed.

A patient was 4 months into treatment. Her rate of weight loss had declined from 2–4 lb (0.9–1.8 kg) per week to 1 lb (0.5 kg) or less. She was at a loss to account for this decline and she attributed it to her "metabolism." The therapist decided that she and the patient needed to go back to first principles to identify the nature of the problem. It seemed that the patient was recording everything she ate and drank, and her calorie calculations appeared accurate. On the other hand, it emerged that she now rarely weighed what she ate. She said that she felt that this was no longer necessary because she now knew the size of her portions. The therapist said that this was probably true but, given the decline in the rate of weight loss, it would be worth reinstituting food weighing for a few weeks to see how accurate her estimates were. This was set up as an experiment. It emerged that, although she was accurate in estimating the weight of some foods (e.g., portions of meat or fish), she was markedly inaccurate in her estimates of others (e.g., pasta). The therapist and patient concluded that this underestimation of portion sizes could well be contributing to the decline in her rate of weight loss. They decided that she should continue to monitor her portion sizes for the meantime. They also noted that the reinstitution of weighing had the added benefit of reducing her food intake (a common phenomenon) with the result that her rate of weight loss returned to its previous level.

3. *Is the patient accurately counting calories?* The quality of calorie counting should also receive detailed attention. Therapists should find out how patients have been using the calorie guide and should ask whether they have any questions about its use. While reviewing the records, therapists should ask patients how they calculated the calorie content of a range of items consumed, starting with easy ones (e.g., items of fruit, packets of food) and moving on to more difficult ones (e.g., restaurant meals). Therapists should be careful to ask these questions in a friendly, interested manner, rather than a challenging fashion. The aim is not to test or judge patients, but to help them improve their accuracy. Where probable inaccuracies are detected, therapists should model how to do the calculation in question or give advice on ways to improve the patient's accuracy of calorie counting. (It is recommended that therapists spend some weeks calculating the calorie content of their own diets so that they appreciate the challenges the task involves).

At one point in reviewing her monitoring records, a patient became uncomfortable. The therapist sensed her discomfort and asked her what was wrong. She admitted that she had not written down everything she had eaten that evening. Her records suggested that she stopped eating at 7.30 P.M., but in fact she had eaten more or less continuously between 8.30 and 10.00 P.M. (an eating pattern sometimes given the pejorative label *grazing*). She was deeply ashamed of the way that she had eaten, and she had decided not to record it. The therapist thanked her for being honest with him. He acknowledged that it is difficult to write down things one feels ashamed about. Through the use of questioning and a nonjudgmental stance, the therapist was able to help the patient see the importance of tackling all her difficulties with eating including those she felt embarrassed about.

Some patients will return having not monitored. The therapist must try to understand why this has happened because it predicts a poor outcome. The explanation should be sought in an accepting but concerned manner. Sometimes it is appropriate to react with an element of surprise, as not monitoring will sabotage treatment. Likely reasons for the failure to monitor need to be addressed. It is important to restate the rationale for monitoring and its importance.

Of course, reluctance to monitor may signify a more general problem with motivation. If this is the case, the procedures described in session 0 should be employed. It is a mistake to ignore signs of poor motivation because they can be the first sign of impending attrition.

After detailed consideration of the *process* of recording, therapists should consider the *content* of the monitoring records. The therapist should review with the patient his or her main source of calories. In doing so the therapist should ask for the patient's view as well as forming his or her own.

It is good practice for therapists to summarize the outcome of the review of the monitoring records, prefacing the summary with an enquiry as to whether this has been a typical week.

Setting the Agenda for the Remainder of the Session

The therapist and patient should next agree on an agenda so that they both know what is planned for the remainder of the session. The patient should be given an opportunity to put items on the agenda (e.g., if they have any questions). In the case of this session (which is atypical to the extent that so much time will have been devoted to the process of recording), the likely agenda items include identifying concerns about treatment, educating about health risks associated with obesity, and starting restricting energy intake.

Identifying Concerns about Treatment.   Therapists should ask patients whether they have any questions or concerns about what has been discussed so far, and these should be discussed. Therapists should stress once again that the distinctive feature of this treatment is its emphasis on long-term weight change.

Educating about Health Risks Associated with Obesity.   Therapists should discuss the health risks associated with obesity in the spirit of informing patients about the condition rather than scaring them. As noted earlier we prefer the expression *being overweight* and believe that it should generally be used in place of *obesity*. A useful starting point is to ask the patient what they already know about the risks associated with being overweight, and then to supplement their knowledge as needed.

The main health risks of obesity are as follows:

- Hypertension (high blood pressure, associated with risk of strokes)
- Cardiovascular disease (coronary artery disease, peripheral vascular disease, heart failure)
- Abnormal blood cholesterol levels (associated with risk of heart disease)
- Diabetes
- Sleep apnea (a condition in which the upper respiratory airways collapse during sleep, resulting in people snoring loudly, waking up suddenly, and then immediately returning to sleep; this can result in severely disrupted sleep with marked daytime tiredness)
- Osteoarthritis (wearing away of the tissue that protects the joints, e.g., knee, hip, and back)

An important point for therapists to convey is that weight loss significantly reduces all these adverse consequences of obesity. Even losing a modest amount of weight (5% of initial body weight) can reduce or eliminate disorders associated with obesity (Blackburn, 2002). For further information about the health risks associated with obesity, see Manson, Skerrett, & Willett (2002) and Pi-Sunyer (2002).

Educating about Unhealthy Methods of Weight Control. Patients who report using self-induced vomiting, laxatives, or diuretics to control their weight should be informed that these methods are ineffective and may have serious health consequences (see Fairburn, 1995).

Introducing an Energy-Restricted Diet. Assuming that the patient has managed to record their calorie intake, a calorie-restricted diet should now be prescribed. A suitable starting level for most patients is an average intake of 1,500 calories daily. In occasional cases the initial calorie level can be set higher, for instance when the patient has a particularly high baseline food intake and a decrease to 1,500 calories daily would probably be too difficult to achieve (i.e., the goal would be unrealistic). Even in these cases, the aim would usually be to move toward a 1,500-calorie-per-day intake as soon as possible.

Some patients will want to decrease their intake to lower than an average of 1,500 calories daily. These patients should be informed that this relatively modest level of calorie restriction is generally appropriate, because in the great majority of cases, it results in weight loss averaging 1–2 lb (0.5–1.0 kg) per week. Fifteen hundred daily calories also allows for an adequate balanced diet to be consumed. In contrast a lower calorie intake is difficult for most people to sustain. It is likely that people who say that they find it easy to adhere to such a limit are underestimating their true calorie intake. It is for this reason that we recommend a starting level of 1,500 calories daily, and, if this proves to be easy for the patient to accomplish, then he or she can decrease further to about 1,200 calories daily.

There are four general points to make to all patients:

1. A diet of 1,500 calories per day will result in weight loss (among people who are overweight).
2. This intake involves moderate rather than extreme dietary restriction. Later on in treatment, further restriction may be worth considering.
3. The key issue is adherence to the dietary restriction. This is greatly assisted by accurate calorie counting.
4. Keeping a running calorie total during the day also helps compliance.

Having introduced the notion of a 1,500-calorie limit, therapists should ask patients for their reaction to the prospect of cutting down their eating in this way. Generally this leads naturally on to a discussion of the patient's ideas as to how he or she might achieve this reduction. It should be stressed that the 1,500-calorie limit is a *guideline* for their average calorie intake. There is nothing magical about this figure, and it does not need to be rigidly followed day by day. On some days the patient may eat somewhat more than this, and on other days he or she may eat somewhat less. The goal is that the patient's *average* daily intake is 1,500 calories (i.e., 10,500 calories per week) without significant day-to-day fluctuations.

Summarizing the Session

The therapist or patient should then summarize the main points covered during the session.

Agreeing on Homework

The therapist and patient should agree on the next weeks' homework. In the great majority of cases, it will be to continue to monitor food intake and restrict calorie intake to an average of 1,500 calories daily. This homework will continue throughout the weight loss part of treatment.

Next Appointment

Our practice is to see the patient in about 7 days.

CHAPTER 4

Module II: Establishing and Maintaining Weight Loss

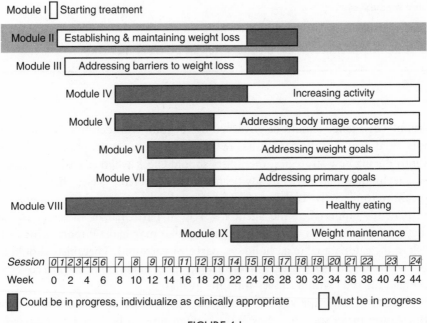

FIGURE 4.1

Once patients are engaged in treatment and have learned to monitor their food and calorie intake, weight loss becomes the goal (see Figure 4.1). This will have been initiated at the end of the previous session (session 1), with the agreement to restrict energy intake to an average of 1,500 calories daily. The goals for this module are twofold:

1. To initiate and maintain weight loss.
2. To determine when to transfer to weight maintenance.

Strategies for achieving these goals are discussed in this chapter.

It has been our practice to hold the first five weight loss sessions (sessions 2–6 inclusive) on a weekly basis, in order to establish the behavior change required. Thereafter sessions become biweekly. Each session should follow a standard format (see Table 4.1), beginning with weighing the patient, reviewing the records and homework, and then setting the agenda for the rest of the

37

TABLE 4.1
―――――
Session Format

1. Record the patient's weight and plot it on the therapist's weight graph. Compare this graph with the patient's. Together the patient and therapist interpret the findings in terms of weight change.

2. Review the latest monitoring records (with the patient taking the lead) together with the patient's success at completing the homework assignments. This is to assess progress and identify issues for inclusion on the agenda.

3. Set agenda collaboratively. Therapists ask patients if there are matters that they want to discuss.

4. Work through the agenda.

5. Devise and agree upon new homework assignments.

6. Summarize the main points covered in the session (by the patient or therapist).

session. The agenda should be governed by the joint considerations of the stage in the treatment that the patient has reached and the review of progress. As well as introducing new strategies, therapists should check whether patients are still using techniques that have already been introduced. Here, as elsewhere, it is important to foster active collaboration between the therapist and patient, inviting the patient's input when the agenda is set. In particular, it is useful to ask whether the patient has any event coming up that may make it more difficult to stick to the calorie goal (e.g., holidays, party, or vacation). Therapists should allow time to discuss such events, while also keeping in mind the need to cover all pertinent material within the session time available.

Working through the agenda should occupy most of these sessions. Therapists should make sure that they leave enough time to both assign homework and provide a summary. Progress should always be highlighted and therapists should do their utmost to ensure that sessions end on a positive note.

When agreeing upon homework with the patient, the principles specified in Table 4.2 should be followed.

Initiating and Maintaining Weight Loss

To achieve weight loss, there must be a sustained energy deficit. This is most easily achieved by reducing intake (in the form of food and drinks). The focus of these treatment sessions is therefore on helping the patient establish and maintain a low energy intake and monitoring the effect this has on their weight. The content of these sessions is presented below. Except where indicated otherwise, these elements should be introduced gradually. Therapists should be careful not to overburden patients with too much information or homework.

TABLE 4.2

Principles for Designing Homework Assignments

- Make the homework relevant to the individual patient, and seek the patient's input.
- Design homework that is specific and achievable.
- Discuss homework sufficiently clearly so that there can be no doubt that patients fully understand what is expected of them.
- Keep amount of homework reasonable, not excessive.
- State a clear rationale for the homework, which the patient understands.
- Expect that homework will be completed.
- Have patients write down the agreed-upon homework, so that it is not forgotten.
- Ask patients to anticipate any difficulty completing homework and address likely obstacles using a problem-solving approach.
- Review the homework at the next treatment session. Praise patients for completing it, and examine any implications arising from the homework at some point in the session. If the homework was not completed, explore the reasons for this. Tackle difficulties using a problem-solving approach.

Weighing the Patient

The therapist should open each session by weighing the patient. This is for two reasons: Most patients will be eager to know their "official" weight, and it provides the therapist with an index of the patient's progress in terms of weight.

After weighing the patient, the therapist should enter the patient's weight on the weight graph. By focusing on trends over time, the patient and therapist can see overall progress. After initiating the 1,500-calorie diet, some immediate weight loss is to be expected. Indeed, the initial rate of weight loss is typically greater than later on.

Having recorded the patient's weight, the therapist should ask the patient about her or his overall progress. The goal is to identify the patient's attitude to their weight loss. At this stage the therapist should simply intervene along the following lines:

- Stress the importance of focusing on weight trends over time (e.g., over the past 3–4 weeks) rather than on single isolated readings. Individual readings cannot be interpreted due to natural day-by-day weight fluctuations and short-term changes in the way the body responds to energy restriction. The occasional week without weight loss is not unusual even in the presence of reasonable behavioral compliance.
- Praise any weight loss.
- Express concern in the face of lack of weight loss if this continues for more than 3 weeks (unless there has been significant weight loss over the previous months but this is now slowing down).
- Stress that the key issue is compliance with the dietary restriction. If there is good adherence to the 1,500-calorie limit, there will be weight loss.

The therapist should repeatedly emphasize that patients need to focus on changing their behavior and if they succeed in doing this their "weight will see to itself."

The following conversation between a patient (P) and her therapist (TH) concerning weight loss illustrates some of these points:

P: So my weight is the same as it was last time then?

TH: Yes. What happened on your scale?

P: About the same. I was hoping something might show on your scale.

TH: How have things been this week?

P: OK—at least I thought things had gone fairly well.

TH: How are the calories looking?

P: I have averaged just below 1,500.

TH: And are you confident that you managed to record everything? Is there any thing you might have missed?

P: No, I'm sure I got everything down—I'm very careful about that. I keep my sheets on my desk at work so I do not miss things during the day.

TH: Great, that is excellent. Are you still managing to weigh everything you eat? Sometimes people feel it is a bit of an effort after they have been doing it a while. Or have there been any occasions this week when you have had to estimate—meals out for example?

P: Yes, I am still weighing food. I do have to estimate meals from the cafeteria at work, but I've been doing that all along. Nothing has changed. Actually I did go out for supper one night, to a friend's house, but I asked her for the recipe so I thought I had made a good estimate from that.

TH: Yes, that is a really good way of working it out—you know exactly what you've had then. Is there anything else you can think of that might have resulted in your being less accurate than normal?

P: No, as I said I thought I had a really good week.

TH: That sounds great. I think it is important that we keep this in perspective. You have lost weight consistently up until now, and if you are sticking to your calories and recording accurately then your weight will undoubtedly continue to decrease. The laws of physics are pretty clear about that—if you take in fewer calories than you use up, you will lose weight! So if you keep doing the right things, your weight will sort itself out.

It might help to remember that everyone's weight shifts up and down throughout the course of the day because of fluid shifts, hormones, and so on. We could weigh you one day and you might be in a "trough"—at the lowest point of one of these shifts—then the next time we weighed you, you could be at a "peak." These day-by-day shifts in weight make it impossible to interpret isolated readings. The way to get round that is to look at your weight over a period of 3–4 weeks. This is why we keep the graph. It is pretty clear from your graph that the overall trend is downward, so if you keep up with the recording, and stick to your calories as you have done, we can be confident that the trend will continue in the right direction.

As in session 1, therapists should also check that patients have weighed themselves once a week at home as agreed. They should have recorded their weight on their personal weight graph. Difficulties with home weighing should be explored and addressed.

Assessing Compliance with the Energy-Restricted Diet

Having addressed patients' progress in terms of weight and weighing, therapists now need to turn to their progress in dietary terms. The point to emphasize is that if they comply with the dietary regimen, weight loss will result. Thus *compliance with the restriction of energy intake should be the primary focus of these sessions.*

It is good practice to start the assessment of compliance by asking patients for their global judgment on how well they have been doing since the last appointment. A general enquiry should suffice. The aim is to get the patient's general, subjective appraisal of their progress. Later, having gone through the monitoring records and assessed compliance, patients should be asked to review their original appraisal of their progress. Many patients will find that they focused on what they have not achieved rather than on what they have accomplished, thereby producing a biased, negative assessment of their progress. This is demoralizing and can lead to the abandonment of their efforts to lose weight. Some patients have the opposite tendency in that they "turn a blind eye" to their difficulties. This is also problematic as it results in their failing to address problems. Poor weight loss in the face of apparent good compliance can be the result of this type of bias. Whatever the direction of the bias, therapists should help patients see the discrepancy and its implications for their views on their competence at weight control. The goal is to help patients get better at accurately appraising their progress.

Reviewing Self-Monitoring

The review of the monitoring records will have taken a considerable portion of session 1. If there were difficulties with the process of self-monitoring (e.g., inaccuracies or problems with calorie calculations), a reasonably thorough review is also indicated in the next few sessions. However, as soon as the patient is complying with self-monitoring without too much difficulty, the review of monitoring records should become briefer (ranging from 5–15 minutes depending on the particular patient and circumstances). The goals of the review are to:

1. check and reinforce continuing compliance with monitoring and other homework assignments;
2. evaluate progress and problems with a view to determining the agenda for the session;
3. identify and reinforce specific changes that the patient has made (this sets a positive tone for the session; it underscores the general emphasis on the patient's strengths and assets rather than on weaknesses or deficits); and
4. identify and reinforce cumulative change.

Therapists should beware of getting sidetracked early on in sessions by focusing on the first problem encountered in the monitoring records (e.g., talking in detail about an episode of binge eating and how it could have been prevented). They should also avoid becoming bogged down in unnecessary detail (e.g., doggedly going through each meal of each day). Both are unsatisfactory and unnecessary because they interfere with the task of identifying priorities for the treatment agenda. They also start the session off on a negative footing, and they take too much time. Instead, the therapist should aim to review the monitoring records relatively briskly to identify the major themes that need to be addressed. For example, a patient may have recorded a number of episodes of overeating. The initial review would not be the time to examine each of these episodes or to begin to intervene with a view to eliminating them. Rather, the therapist should overtly flag them so that the patient knows that they will be addressed later in the session, at which point one or two selected examples will become the focus of attention.

It is always important to praise patients. Good monitoring and calorie counting deserve strong praise. Both are demanding tasks, and it is extremely tempting to cut corners. This is particularly likely later on in treatment when recording has lost its novelty and can seem more of a chore than anything else. At this point praise may be particularly important to help patients continue with their weight loss efforts.

Establishing a Collaborative Style

Throughout this process the therapist should have a concerned, nonjudgmental, and collaborative attitude. The goal is that the therapist and patient *together* try to assess progress and solve problems. It is especially important not to be confrontational as this can undermine compliance rather than improve it. Example 1, below, lacks a collaborative approach, whereas example 2 illustrates collaboration.

Example 1: Lack of Collaboration between Therapist (TH) and Patient (P)

P: That was a terrible day! I had one cookie then I just could not stop. I ended up eating most of the package. I wasn't hungry, but I just needed something.

TH: Maybe you could try fruit instead of cookies if you feel you need a snack?

P: I suppose I could give that a try.

[The patient is unlikely to have felt satisfied with this encounter and may be even more unlikely to change his or her behavior as a result of it. The therapist did not foster a collaborative approach. Jumping in with solutions without first specifying the problem is rarely helpful.]

Example 2: Collaboration between Therapist (TH) and Patient (P)

P: That was a terrible day! I had one cookie then I just could not stop. I ended up eating most of the package. I wasn't hungry, but I just needed something.

TH: How did you feel afterwards?

P: Well, I felt better for a while. The cookies tasted really good! But later I felt awful—guilty and stupid.

TH: Can you tell me a bit more about what happened before you ate those cookies?

P: I have not been sleeping well lately, so I was really tired. Then my husband started complaining that dinner wasn't ready. He doesn't seem to notice that I work too, and our daughter had to be taken to her music lesson, there was just no way I could fit all that in. We ended up having an argument. Then I ate those cookies.

TH: What were you thinking just before you ate them?

P: I was really upset. I never get any time for myself. I'm like the family servant.

TH: So you were feeling upset, and that you need time for yourself . . . maybe that you need looking after too?

P: That's right.

TH: Can you remember what you were thinking after you had eaten the first few cookies?

P: I was thinking, "Blow this diet business! I need these or I'll go crazy!"

TH: But you ended up feeling bad about eating them?

P: Yes, but not right away. While I was eating, I really enjoyed those cookies.

TH: So eating seems to help temporarily but makes you feel bad later on?

P: Yes, I get upset when I think I've blown my chances of losing weight.

TH: It sounds like eating those cookies was one way of making a bit of space for yourself; asserting your right to do things just for you. But in the end, it leaves you feeling worse and hampers your weight loss efforts. Maybe we could think about other ways of coping when you feel frustrated or upset? Do you think that would be worth a try?

P: Yes, I guess so.

[The therapist worked more collaboratively here. He asked many more questions, getting the patient to work out why she ate the cookies. He listened carefully and fed back to the patient to make sure he was understanding correctly. Solutions developed as a result of a collaborative analysis of problems are likely to be more effective than formulaic solutions arrived at with little or no collective thought. It is always best to ask questions before leaping in with answers].

Maximizing Adherence to the Dietary Regimen

The therapist should praise adherence to the dietary regimen (as judged by patient's recording of his or her behavior, not on the basis of the patient's latest weight, although the trend in weight change over several weeks should also be considered). All aspects of compliance should be identified and praised. Partial successes (such as eating less than normal when eating out, even if the 1,500-calorie goal was exceeded) should also receive the therapist's attention. The therapist should be encouraging and enthusiastic. On the other hand, if the patient's progress seems precarious, then potential sources of difficulty need to be identified and addressed along the lines specified in Chapter 5.

One difficulty arises when there is no weight loss over a period of several weeks, despite apparent compliance. Under these circumstances there is no escaping the fact that the patient's energy intake must be higher than it appears. On a 1,500-calorie diet, all patients with obesity should lose weight. This should be explained to the patients so as to avoid their attributing problems to their physiology (e.g., "I just have a slow metabolism"). Instead, a thorough review of their energy intake is needed in order to detect the various possible sources of inaccuracy (see Chapter 5).

To help patients adhere to the 1,500-calorie goal, the following three strategies should be recommended:

1. *Have a plan for the day.* The patient should have a good idea what and when they will be eating during the day. This can be written on the back of the day's monitoring record.
2. *Keep a running calorie total throughout the day,* to monitor progress toward the calorie target. This running total should be noted on the monitoring record.
3. *Be on the alert for potential problems.* For example, if patients are aware that they will be going out for a meal and it will be difficult to keep within their usual limit, they should think in advance about how they will deal with this problem. In general they will need to take one or both of two courses of action:

   a. Develop a definite plan for dealing with the meal itself to minimize the risk of excessive consumption.
   b. Compensate for any increase in intake. Eating less than usual earlier in the day is risky because it can lead to feelings of deprivation and hunger, which may encourage subsequent overeating. Eating a little less on several other days in the week (e.g., eating 1,400 kcal/day the 2 days before and 2 days after eating out) is wiser. It is also consistent with the goal of maintaining an average intake, over the course of the week,

of 1,500 calories daily. On the other hand, major oscillations in the patient's calorie intake are not to be encouraged. It is our practice to advise patients to aim to keep within 300 calories of the 1,500-calorie target (i.e., a range of 1,200–1,800 kcal/day).[1]

In general, when the therapist detects problems with the patient's adherence, these should be addressed following the guidelines in Chapter 5.

To help patients identify meals and snacks that are compatible with the calorie limit, therapists should suggest that they look through low-fat/low-calorie recipe books for ideas. Books that specify the calories per portion are the most useful. Looking through the calorie book itself is also worthwhile. Of course, patients will want to construct meals and snacks of their own, and this should be encouraged. One useful strategy is for patients to identify days that went particularly well and to repeat meals and snacks eaten on these days. The goal is that patients build up a repertoire of meals and snacks that they like.

A patient found that she was tempted to buy high-calorie foods on her way home from work, as she felt hungry and knew it would be at least an hour before she got home and could start preparing her meal. By taking extra fruit with her to work, which she could eat on the bus on the way home, she was able to resist buying snacks for herself.

Artificial sweeteners can help some people adhere to the calorie-restricted diet. In our experience they are most relevant to the following groups of people:

- Those who consume large quantities of soft drinks (soda)
- Those who take sugar in their coffee or tea
- Those who eat stewed fruit

In such cases the patient should be told that trying to limit sugar intake will assist in weight loss. However, because it is not realistic to try to change a long-standing liking for sweet foods, therapists should work with patients in finding a way to limit their sugar intake while accepting their preference for sweet foods. In this context artificial sweeteners have a role and should be mentioned.

Establishing Adherence to the Principles of Healthy Eating

The patient's adherence to the calorie-restricted diet should conform to the principles of healthy eating. Four issues need to be considered: temporal pattern of eating, food choice, eating style, and cognitive aspects of eating.

---

[1] Some patients eat too little at times. This is not a good idea because it encourages overeating at other times. Patients who want to eat fewer than 1,500 calories a day should be advised that their intake should not fall below 1,200 calories daily and that it might well be more difficult to maintain this level of restriction.

Temporal Pattern of Eating

The patient should eat at regular intervals through the day (generally three meals and one or more planned snacks) without "picking" at food outside these planned times. A pattern of regular eating helps to reduce the risk of overeating.

Evening snacks are especially important as many people have difficulty controlling their eating in the evening. Often this difficulty stems from an attempt not to eat after the evening meal. The trouble with this goal is that it leads to feelings of deprivation at the very time when patients are most at risk of overeating as they tend to be at home with easy access to food. Therapists should recommend that patients plan an appetizing evening snack, making an allowance for this in their daily calorie allowance. To minimize feelings of deprivation, this snack should be a highlight in the day's eating (i.e., something to look forward to).

A patient liked to eat a snack in the evening, and therefore decided to distribute her calorie allowance so that it would allow for this. The therapist encouraged this on the grounds that regular eating and planned snacks are important to avoid feelings of deprivation. This patient had been used to eating large amounts of nuts or chocolate for snacks and felt it was likely that she might experience feelings of deprivation and frustration if she had to eat "diet food" for a snack. The therapist suggested that the patient compile a list of foods that were of "high value" to her. The patient and therapist then reviewed these foods to see which might form calorie-controlled snacks. Several possibilities presented themselves; for example, "special" fruit, such as pineapple or strawberries, or calorie- and portion-controlled chilled desserts, such as mousse. The patient therefore bought these foods so that her evening snack was "luxurious" as well as compatible with her calorie goal.

Food Choice

The patient should eat a broad range of foods. This is important both for health reasons and to protect against binge eating (as excluding foods encourages some people to binge eat). The therapist should introduce the notion of "less food, but good food." It is worthwhile encouraging some patients to use some of the money that they will save by eating less to buy more expensive—and perhaps novel—food. No foods should be banned.

All patients should be asked to identify which foods contribute most to their calorie intake, and then helped to see that foods containing the largest number of calories per unit weight are those that are high in fat (i.e., they are "energy dense"). This information should be used to initiate a discussion of the relative energy densities of protein, fat, and carbohydrate (and alcohol). The following points should be made:

• For the purpose of weight control, a calorie is a calorie. One hundred calories of carrots is the same as 100 calories of whipped cream. However, by adjusting food choices and taking particular note of the relative energy (calorie) densities of different foods, patients can find calorie-restricted diets more satisfying and thereby easier to follow.

• Fat is considerably more energy dense than protein or carbohydrate. Fat has more than twice as many calories per gram of weight than protein or carbohydrate. There are 9 calories in each gram of fat, but only 4 calories in each gram of protein or carbohydrates. Therefore, if patients substitute some of their fat intake with carbohydrate or protein, they will be able to eat more food. This discussion of energy density will make most sense to patients if the therapist focuses on foods rather than macronutrients. Therefore therapists should use illustrative foods whenever possible, choosing foods that the particular patient tends to eat. Some patients may point out that starchy foods— such as bread, cereal, rice, and pasta—can contribute a considerable number of calories. Although this is true if they are eaten in significant amounts, the point is that they are considerably more filling than high-fat foods.

• Limiting fat intake also has the major benefit of reducing some of the health risks associated with obesity (particularly that of cardiovascular disease).

If the patient is eating a high-fat diet and this is proving a barrier to weight loss, the therapist should introduce Module VIII ("Healthy Eating") at this point.

Eating Style

Patients should pay attention to how they eat. Whenever possible, eating should be planned and formalized, even if this seems artificial. Patients should be encouraged to decide what they will eat and drink in advance and make sure it is all laid out. It is helpful if meals are eaten in a set place at home and the patient is sitting down. Food should be savored rather than eaten automatically so that the patient gets the full "value" out of what they are eating. Otherwise the patients may find that they have finished their meal or snack without having really noticed eating it.

Cognitive Aspects of Eating

Patients should be encouraged to see that the way one thinks about food and eating is also important. For example, people who diet rigidly with many rules about how they should eat are prone to react in an extreme fashion to any breaking of their rules, however minor. Flexible dieting in which there are guidelines rather than rules is much less likely to result in problems of this type (see Chapter 5 for how to address this issue if it appears to be a problem).

TABLE 4.3
─────────

Information for Patients on Energy Balance

───

ENERGY BALANCE

The key points
- To have a stable weight, your energy intake (what you eat as food and drink) must equal the energy you burn up (that needed to keep your body processes going and for physical activity).
- Weight problems develop when your energy intake (calories) exceeds the energy you are burning up over a sustained period of time.
- This positive energy balance (excess energy) is stored in the body mainly as fat.
- Excess weight (fat) is only lost when you create a negative energy balance so that your body draws on its energy (fat) stores.
- A sustained reduction in your energy intake (as food and drink) is needed to produce weight loss.
- In principle your rate of weight loss could be accelerated by increasing the energy you burn up as a result of physical activity, but in practice the additional benefits are not great. On the other hand, regular physical activity does help weight maintenance.
- Once you reach your target weight range, you will need to adjust your eating and activity level to stabilize your weight. This is an important skill that requires practice.

Why do some people develop weight problems?
- There are two main reasons and often they both apply:
  - Eating too much (energy intake too high)
  - Not being active enough (not burning enough energy)
- Metabolic, hormonal, or other medical problems are rarely relevant, although people vary somewhat in the amount of energy their body needs to keep running.
- Weight problems tend to run in families. This can be due to the family environment or to genetic factors or both.
- Genes have a definite influence on body weight, so if you come from a family in which many people have significant weight problems, you are likely to be genetically vulnerable to similar difficulties.
- Psychological factors lead some people to overeat. Some people overeat in response to stress or when they are unhappy or bored, whereas others find that their appetite is diminished. Extreme dieting can also encourage overeating.
- Poor eating habits can also be learned (at home, school or work, or due to other circumstances). A particular problem in our society today is that most people eat too much high-fat food, largely because it is readily available and tastes good.
- As a society we are also much less active than we used to be. Many people have jobs that involve little activity and people are also much less active at home.

───

Educating about Weight Regulation

At some point in the weight loss process, patients should be educated about the principles of weight regulation (energy balance). The topic should be introduced by explaining that it is important for the patient to understand how difficulties with weight control develop and what can be done to counteract them. The information should be kept simple and to the point. Table 4.3 shows the points to cover. These are also listed in Handout E, which the therapist should go over with the patient.

Therapists should emphasize the positive aspect of this information by explaining that, although a number of the factors discussed may make patients vulnerable to weight problems, there is no reason to believe that they cannot successfully change their weight. Therapists should remind patients that they can lose weight if they adjust their energy balance so that the amount of energy they use up is greater than the amount of energy provided by the food they are consuming. The most effective way of doing this is to consume less energy in the form of food and drink, and this is why the focus is on helping them change their eating and drinking habits. Therapists should acknowledge that restricting one's intake is hard work, especially as it often involves changing deeply in-grained habits, and patients generally live in an environment that encourages the consumption of high-fat food. In this regard, therapists should draw the patient's attention to the wide availability of food, to the great choice that exists, and to the ready availability of highly palatable high-fat foods (e.g., fast food). They should also point out that eating is often a social activity with many social occasions and celebrations revolving around eating out or in the home. In addition to these ubiquitous pressures to eat, patients may have learned as children to eat large portions, to finish everything on the plate (whether they were hungry or not), and to use eating as a means of regulating their mood. Therapists should discuss in detail those pressures that seem most relevant to the individual patient.

Introducing Weekly Reviews

Patients may need help in adjusting to changes in appointment frequency. As explained earlier, our practice is to hold weekly appointments for the first 6 weeks, and then to hold appointments every 2 weeks. Two sessions before reducing the frequency of appointments, we ask patients to predict difficulties that might arise as a result. In addition, they are advised to hold weekly "review sessions" with themselves. On weeks in which there is no session with the therapist, these reviews can serve as substitute appointments and a time for "taking stock." On weeks in which there is an appointment, the review serves as valuable preparation for the forthcoming session.

Review sessions should be formal, scheduled ahead, and given priority, just as if they were an appointment with the therapist. To explain their purpose and how to conduct them, the therapist should go over information in Table 4.4, which is also reproduced in Handout F. At each subsequent appointment, therapists should ask patients about their most recent review sessions, their own appraisal of their progress, and the homework that they set for themselves. Some patients may choose to involve others (e.g., a supportive spouse or friend) in their review sessions.

A patient initially used weekly reviews effectively, taking care to identify what she had achieved, and setting herself aims for the week as well as examining what had not gone well. However, her weight loss became slower, although she was still apparently compliant. She felt frustrated,

TABLE 4.4

Information for Patients on Conducting Review Sessions

REVIEW SESSIONS

Now that your appointments will be at 2-week intervals, it is important to have weekly, between-session, appointments with yourself. This might seem odd but it can be extremely valuable. The purpose of these review sessions is to ensure that you remain alert to your progress and any problems that you might be having. They also help you maintain momentum between our sessions.

These review sessions are important and should be given priority. It is best to schedule them in advance just like a treatment appointment. It is helpful if each session has the following structure:

- Review of your progress based on your most recent monitoring records and any change in your weight. In doing this you should take account of the "homework" that was agreed at the last session.
- Identify everything that you have achieved over the last week. It is important to give yourself credit for your achievements.
- Set yourself one or two specific goals for the forthcoming week.

It is also very important to continue to weigh yourself at weekly intervals and record your weight on your graph.

At each appointment we will discuss how you have managed with the review and the goals that you set yourself.

Making a habit of assessing your progress in this way will prepare you for the future when you will no longer be coming for treatment.

---

and her weekly reviews became negative in tone. The therapist helped her to see that even though her weight had not decreased, she had made (and sustained) other important behavioral changes, which were worth noting. The therapist also explained that it is important to look for positive aspects of the week gone by, as focusing solely on negative aspects gives an unbalanced view of progress and can precipitate a slide into thoughts of failure and being unable to cope. The patient identified with this and was careful in future to include positive features in her reviews. This helped her to adhere to the treatment even when things were going less well than she would have liked.

An example of a balanced review is given below:

I have not lost any weight this week but I know this happens some weeks, even when I have adhered to my calorie limit and eaten healthily. I feel that I have done pretty well at sticking to my goal this week. I did especially well at the buffet, when I used the strategies I had planned. I do still feel low in spirits but I am coping, and I am not comfort eating. My aim for the next week is to use my exercise video twice. I feel a bit sluggish, and I think exercising will help me feel more positive and energized (and it will use up a few extra calories!).

Identifying and Encouraging Changes in Domains Other Than Eating

At about monthly intervals from week 6 onwards, therapists should ask patients about any changes they have experienced or made in domains of life other than eating and weight. The aim is to broaden the patient's perspective on the benefits that can result as a consequence of treatment, as most patients are primarily weight focused. If successful, this will facilitate the moderation of the patient's weight goals later on in treatment (see Chapter 8).

Any positive changes that appear to be attributable to treatment should be highlighted and praised. Also, if the patient is considering making constructive lifestyle changes (e.g., socializing more or going swimming), these should be strongly encouraged.

> P: I was disappointed by what the scale was telling me, but from the way my clothes are fitting, I can tell there is a change overall.
>
> TH: That sounds good. Do you feel different in any other ways?
>
> P: Yes, I do, I feel a lot better. I have got more energy. I am less tired. And I have bought some new clothes.
>
> TH: How did that go?
>
> P: It went well. I bought a new skirt, a different color from what I normally get, and a new blouse. I wore them when we went out, and I got lots of compliments!
>
> TH: Wonderful! So several things have changed even though you are not losing weight as fast as you would like?
>
> P: Yes, I guess so.
>
> TH: Well that is excellent. It is really important to identify these sorts of changes and not just to think about the number on the scale, so it is great that you have noticed all these things.

Addressing Eating Out, Vacations, and Special Occasions

Eating out, vacations, and other special occasions pose particular challenges for those trying to restrict their calorie intake. As with most aspects of weight control, planning ahead is crucial.

Tables 4.5, 4.6, and 4.7 (also reproduced as Handouts G, H, and I) outline complementary behavioral and cognitive strategies to help patients deal with these situations. Using this information as a guide, patients should be helped to plan their own individual strategies to cope with such circumstances. In general patients should be encouraged to consider whether they regard eating large quantities of food as an essential part of vacations and special occasions. If they do, the therapist should briefly explore their reasons for this and whether a different attitude might be more helpful. Patients should be helped to find out whether there are features of social occasions or vacations, other than eating

TABLE 4.5

Information for Patients on Eating in Social Situations

SOCIAL EATING

Eating out or with other people can pose additional challenges when you are trying to control your calorie intake. Planning ahead is important. In particular, it is helpful to ensure that you have thought about how to deal with both the practical issues related to social eating and your attitude to keeping to your calorie limit. Most situations can be successfully tackled if you have a plan for dealing with them. On the other hand, if you are caught unawares you are at greater risk of experiencing problems.

Here are some specific tips for dealing with eating out.

A. Practical Strategies

General

- Plan far enough in advance, as you may want to adjust your eating in the days before (and/or after) the event to "bank" calories. You will often also need to plan a strategy to deal with the specific situation (see below).
- Think about the difficulties you will encounter. Consider the following:
  - The amounts and types of food that will be provided
  - Social pressures to eat
  - The availability of "extras" (e.g., premeal appetizers, after-dinner chocolates)
  - Alcohol
- It may be useful to think about how you have dealt with similar situations in the past.

In all the situations mentioned below it is helpful to plan in advance. This gives you time to anticipate any difficulties that might arise and how to cope with them. Here are some practical tips that may help. Note that not all will suit you or the situation.

Restaurants

- Participate in the choice of restaurant if possible; look at the menu in advance, or possibly telephone the restaurant to ask about availability of low-fat or low-calorie dishes.
- If possible, ask for food to be served without extra butter, and for dressings and sauces to be served separately so you can control the amount you have. Consider asking for a smaller portion of the main dish with extra vegetables or salad.
- Be wary of set menus. They may include dishes that are not good choices for people who are trying to lose weight, but are also difficult to resist when you have already paid for them.
- Try asking for fresh fruit as a dessert, or maybe share a dessert with somebody else.

Buffets

- Look carefully at what is available before you actually put anything on your plate. Identify a few foods that you would really enjoy (rather than trying a bit of everything) and choose some low-calorie options such as salad or rice to fill you up.
- Try using a side plate rather than a full-size dinner plate.
- Treat it as you would a sit-down meal. Visit the buffet table only once, and then when you have eaten get rid of your plate as soon as possible.
- Alternatively, ask someone else to bring you some food, and tell them what you would like.

Entertaining in Your Own Home

- Consider whether you are obliged to provide a high-fat, high-calorie meal. Many people are either watching their weight or being careful about their diet for health reasons. A lower-fat meal is just as likely to be welcomed by guests and certainly does not indicate poor hospitality.
- Single-portion foods, such as individual chicken pieces, are often easier to manage and avoid the difficulty of having tempting leftovers.

continued

TABLE 4.5

(continued)

- If you do have food left over, either give it to guests to take with them or freeze it immediately.
- If you tend to pick while preparing food, try immersing used dishes and utensils immediately in soapy water or chewing gum while you cook.

Eating at Someone Else's House

- If possible, try to find out in advance what will be served. If you know the host/hostess well, consider contacting them in advance to explain your situation and ask if it would be possible for him or her to help. You could perhaps find out what he or she is planning to serve so that you can decide in advance what you will eat, and plan your day accordingly.
- It may be possible to offer to take a dish with you, so that you know there will be at least one low-calorie option.
- Offer to help serve so that you can control your portion size, or ask for a small portion.
- Fill your plate with salad or vegetables, and take only small amounts of high-calorie dishes. This helps to control the calories and avoids drawing attention to your weight control efforts.
- Asking for recipes may be a good (and socially acceptable) way of finding out what went into a meal so as to calculate the calories you consumed.

B. Other Issues

Pressure to Eat

If you tend to feel under pressure to eat more than you had planned, try to work out exactly what makes you feel this way. Are you concerned that people will be offended if you do not eat everything you are offered, or that you will draw attention to yourself if you do not eat as much as everyone else? If you can work out precisely what the problem is, it will be easier to think of ways to cope. For example, if you are concerned that your host will be offended if you do not eat much, you might decide it would be helpful to practice saying "No" politely but firmly. You could test out whether politely declining foods is likely to cause offence. You might do this by thinking about how you would feel if you were the host and someone declined food in this way; or by watching carefully to see if other people always eat large portions of everything available, and how others react if they do not. If you are concerned about drawing attention to yourself by not doing what everyone else is doing, you might observe the reactions of others to people who, for example, are not drinking alcohol, perhaps because they are driving, or perhaps simply because it is their preference not to do so. Ask yourself whether you think it would be reasonable to react negatively to such situations and whether you would do so.

Feeling Deprived

Although planning ahead to make the most of your calories is helpful, it is not uncommon to feel that social events revolve entirely around high-calorie food and drink and to think that not being able to eat or drink everything that you would like will make these events less enjoyable. You could test this view to see whether you really enjoy occasions less if you limit your food and alcohol. Also, you could try focusing on all those nonfood aspects of social events that make them enjoyable (e.g., talking to friends, having time to relax, not having to wash the dishes) so that food and drink become less important aspects of social events.

Coping with Unexpected Occasions

Sometimes invitations to eat arrive unexpectedly—someone drops in and suggests having lunch together, or friends come around with take-out, or somebody suggests going for a meal after a movie. It is helpful to take a few minutes to think clearly about how to handle the situation. You may decide to join in with the meal, and cut down on calories later in the day or the next day. Alternatively, if you have already eaten or planned what you are going to eat, you may need to respond differently: perhaps by suggesting another time when you could have a meal together or explaining that you will just have a small amount as you have already eaten. You may wish to experiment with different possibilities and find out which one works best for you.

TABLE 4.6

Information for Patients on Planning for Vacations

PLANNING FOR VACATIONS

Vacations can pose additional challenges when you are trying to control your calorie intake. You may be in unfamiliar surroundings where the food choice may be quite different from home, and you may have less control than usual over the preparation of food.

Planning ahead is important. In particular, it is helpful to ensure that you have thought about how to deal with both the practical issues related to eating, as well as how you might feel about keeping to a calorie limit. Most situations can be successfully tackled if you have a plan for dealing with them. On the other hand, if you are caught unawares you are at greater risk of encountering problems.

General

Vacations are a time to relax and enjoy yourself, and sometimes people see this as incompatible with restricting their consumption of food and drink. It is worth considering how you can make the most of your vacation without undoing all the hard work you have put into losing weight. The first step is to decide on your goal over the vacation. Do you want to continue losing weight or to maintain your current weight? If you intend to stick to your calorie goal with the aim of continuing to lose weight, be clear and realistic about how you will achieve this goal. If you think that it is not realistic to stick to your calorie goal, it may be best to work out a slightly higher calorie limit with your therapist for the vacation period, with the aim of maintaining your weight.

In making decisions about your goals, it may be helpful to consider what, besides being able to drink and eat freely, will be enjoyable about the time away. A vacation may provide an ideal opportunity to practice the new habits you have learned and experiment with the possibility that you can have an enjoyable time while still limiting your intake of food and alcohol.

Here are some specific practical issues to consider when planning ahead.

Monitoring Food and Weight

- Will you monitor your food and weight while you are away? If so, how? Will scales be available for weighing food and for checking your weight?
- When will you do your weekly reviews? Can you set aside a time with yourself? Would it be helpful to send (fax or E-mail) your weekly reviews to your therapist while you are away?

Arrangements for Travel

- How long will your journey take from door to door? What meals would you normally eat during this time? Will you be traveling overnight or on a long-haul flight? If so, how this might affect your eating pattern?
- What food will be available? Is it worth taking your own to ensure you have control over what you eat? Are you likely to be tempted by the availability of snack foods in gas stations, airports, or trains? Will your food choice be determined by circumstances (e.g., food on an airplane)? If so, would it be worthwhile ordering a special meal?
- What time will it be when you arrive at your destination (and at home on your return journey)? Can you arrange for suitable food to be available (e.g., by leaving a meal in the freezer at home)?
- How can you make it easy to keep monitoring while you travel? Many people find it is difficult to resume monitoring after a gap, so working out how to monitor through unusual situations is worthwhile. Making sure you have your monitoring sheets handy is important, and calculating in advance anything you take with you can make monitoring easier during the journey.

General Arrangements When Away

- Will food be provided? Will you be eating out, preparing your own food, or a combination of these? How will you cope with the particular arrangements? Do you anticipate any difficulties? Planning ahead is likely to be helpful in these situations.
- How will your requirements fit in with the rest of the party?
- What types of food will be available?

Alcohol

- Does your alcohol intake tend to increase when on vacation? How do you intend to manage this?

TABLE 4.7
───────

Information for Patients on Coping with Special Occasions

SPECIAL OCCASIONS

Controlling your calorie intake on special occasions (such as parties, birthdays, weddings, and other celebrations) can be difficult. Such occasions provide a good opportunity to practice the new habits you are learning and to experiment with the possibility of having an enjoyable time without eating too much. This handout summarizes many of the strategies that we recommend for coping with special occasions. It also suggests new and different ways to think about the role of food on special occasions.

Goals

It is generally best to stick to your usual weekly calorie goal (as an average over the week). Be clear and realistic about how you will achieve this. Eating nothing all day in anticipation of a party is likely to lead to overeating later on. Instead, eating lightly the day before or after may be a better plan. Completely avoiding food that you like may also be a mistake. It is usually a good idea to plan to eat such food and incorporate it into your day's eating plan.

Plan Ahead

The single most important strategy for dealing with any special occasion is planning ahead. This is especially important if there will be extra food around over a period of several days, and if there will be more than one special meal or party. High-calorie foods and alcoholic drinks often seem to be an integral part of these events, so it is especially important that you make plans to deal with these challenges. It is generally helpful to make a plan for each day, and you may need to plan several days in advance when celebrations go on for several days.

Monitor

It is very important to continue to monitor. This will keep you informed about how your strategies are working and help you to adjust your plans as necessary. It will also help you to keep focused on your goals.

Alcohol

It is especially important to have a plan for dealing with alcohol; not only does it add calories, but it tends to weaken the resolve to eat moderately.

Focus on Other Pleasurable Aspects of Special Occasions

Although many social events may seem to center on high-calorie food and drinks, consider whether it is possible to celebrate without consuming these in large quantities. It may be helpful to think about ways of making celebrations enjoyable that do not involve eating (or at least eating large quantities of food) and trying these out. Try paying particular attention to the features of social occasions that make them enjoyable. This may lead you to conclude that eating moderate quantities of food would not spoil your enjoyment. Some people even discover that they enjoy occasions more when they eat and drink less.

Dealing with Pressure to Eat

You may feel under pressure to eat more than you had planned. This can happen for many reasons: The sheer abundance of food may tempt you; you may feel people will be offended if you do not eat much; or you may feel that you will be 'the odd one out' if you do not join others in eating and drinking all that is offered. It is always easier to cope with such situations if you have made a plan in advance. Also it is helpful to practice refusing food politely but firmly. You do not have to eat to please others, and people rarely notice what you are eating and drinking.

continued

TABLE 4.7

(continued)

Gifts of Food

On special occasions people may buy chocolate, sweets, cake, or other food for you. If this is likely, would it be worth asking them to buy something else instead? If you feel you could not make this request yourself, perhaps your partner or a relative or friend could discreetly advise others that you would prefer not to be given food. Also it would be helpful to consider how to cope if you receive such food unexpectedly. Could you give it to someone else?

Snacks

Sometimes on special occasions there is a wide variety of snacks on display. Having bowls of nuts, chocolates, and other high-calorie snacks is likely to be a temptation beyond most people's endurance, so plan how best to cope with this situation. When such situations are under your control, you may decide to do things differently.

If you are having to provide snacks:
- Plan the shopping carefully and limit the amount of extra food bought.
- Keep snacks in sealed containers, and only set out small quantities for specific occasions.
- Have alternative, lower-calorie snacks such as raw vegetables with low-calorie dip, fruit, plain (unsweetened or unbuttered) popcorn, and bread sticks.
- The strategies suggested in Handout G on social eating are also relevant to many special occasions.

---

and drinking, that make them enjoyable and whether their level of enjoyment is substantially affected by what they eat.

The Issue of Activity Level and Exercise

Many weight loss treatments place great emphasis on getting patients to be more active, and some advocate strenuous exercise regimens. There are reasons to question the value of this approach:

- Increasing activity levels has a relatively modest effect on energy balance compared with dietary restriction.
- Some patients with obesity find exercise programs aversive. They may be embarrassed by the physical exposure involved, they may feel ashamed about their appearance and performance, and they may find many forms of exercise too physically demanding.
- Adhering to the energy-restricted diet and dealing with obstacles to adherence (see Chapter 5) is already demanding even without additional behavioral goals such as regular exercising. If too many goals are set, there is a risk that in practice few will be met.

This treatment's stance on activity and exercise is to delay focusing on them until consistent weight loss has been established (see Chapter 6). Attention to activity is probably especially important in the later stages of treatment because activity levels have been shown to predict long-term weight maintenance. Of course, patients should not be discouraged from being physically active earlier on in treatment. If they are already active, they should be praised. If they want to take up a new form of activity, they should be encouraged to do so as long as it will not interfere with dietary compliance. Guidelines for encouraging physical activity are provided in Chapter 6.

Early in treatment a patient expressed an interest in increasing her level of physical activity. She was losing weight steadily and making good progress generally. The therapist was encouraging, but did not push the patient to make any concrete plans about exercise. Over the next few sessions, the patient talked about an exercise class that her friend attended, saying she had been invited to go along too. The patient was a little uncertain initially, but over time decided she would try it out, and she set a date to go. The therapist was positive about her plans, and about the benefits of exercise generally.

At the session after the exercise class, the patient appeared distressed. She had found it an aversive experience. Physically the session had been demanding, and she had found it upsetting to watch herself and the other class participants in the mirror, as she saw herself as bigger and clumsier than the others. The therapist listened to the patient's concerns and asked her what she thought she would do. The patient said she was not going to return to the exercise class. The therapist did not press the issue further, and explained that physical activity was an important topic that they would return to later in treatment. She also noted the patient's distress at comparing her body with others, and decided that this would be addressed when they addressed the topic of body image concerns.

Developing Problem-Solving Skills

All patients should be taught problem solving. This skill helps them deal with the types of day-to-day difficulties that face those trying to restrict their food intake. The approach used is derived from the work of Goldfried (D'Zurilla & Goldfried, 1971; Goldfried & Goldfried, 1975).

Ideally it is best to start the training in problem solving by identifying a recent difficulty—for example, an episode of overeating that was precipitated by an external event. Then, using this problem as an example, the therapist should teach the patient the principles of problem solving. The therapist should explain that although many problems may seem overwhelming at first, if they are approached systematically, they usually turn out to be manageable. Acquiring problem-solving skills helps the patient tackle day-to-day difficulties so that they do not lead to overeating.

In principle, effective problem-solving follows these six commonsense steps, together with a final review step:

Step 1. The problem should be identified as soon as possible.

Step 2. The problem should be specified accurately: What exactly is the problem? Rephrasing the problem is often helpful. It may emerge that there are two or more coexisting problems, in which case the following steps should be followed for each problem separately.

Step 3. All ways of dealing with the problem should be considered. The patient should generate as many potential solutions as possible (which is known as "brainstorming"). Some solutions may immediately seem nonsensical or impracticable. Nevertheless, they should be included in the list of possible alternatives. The more solutions that are generated, the more likely a good one will emerge.

Step 4. The likely effectiveness and feasibility of each solution should be thought through, perhaps by drawing up a separate pros and cons list for each solution identified.

Step 5. The best solution or combination of solutions should be selected.

Step 6. The steps required to carry out the chosen solution should be defined, and the solution should be acted upon.

Afterward (usually the following day), the patient should evaluate the entire problem-solving process. This is a crucial step as the goal is not simply to resolve the specific problem in question; rather, it is to become skilled at problem solving. The patient should therefore review each of the steps of the problem-solving process, and consider how it could have been improved.

Having stressed the importance of effective problem solving and explained the steps involved, the therapist should go over these steps using the example problem to demonstrate how the patient should apply problem solving to future difficulties. If time allows, another recent problem should be identified and approached in the same way but with the patient taking the lead. Then, as homework, the patient should be asked to practice problem solving whenever the opportunity arises. To help patients remember the six problem-solving steps, they should be given Handout J. When any difficulty occurs or is foreseen, they should write "problem" in the right-hand column of their monitoring sheet, and then on the back work through the problem-solving steps. They should be told that their problem-solving skills will improve with practice, and that the technique may be applied to any day-to-day difficulty.

In subsequent sessions the therapist should review in detail the patient's attempts at problem solving and suggest improvements as appropriate. It is important to keep in mind that the goal is not solving individual problems, although this is obviously desirable, but rather acquiring and refining problem-solving skills.

A patient planned to go on a camping weekend with a group of friends, and she thought this might be a problem. She worked through the problem-solving steps as follows:

Step 1: Identify the problem early.
How am I going to manage the camping weekend with my friends?

Step 2: Specify the problem accurately.
The problem is that I am at risk of going well over my calorie goal on the camping weekend. This is because:

1. The type of food available on the campsite is high in calories (burgers, etc.).
2. Smelling and seeing all the food tempts me to eat more, and so does seeing the others eat freely.
3. I usually feel more hungry when I am outside and getting more exercise
4. Everyone will be drinking and I will want to join them, but alcohol adds further calories and makes me less careful about what I eat.

Step 3: Consider possible solutions.
1. Tell friends I have decided not to go.
2. Eat nothing all day to save up calories for the main evening meal and then eat and drink like everyone else.
3. Take my own low-calorie food with me in a cooler. Only eat food I have brought and refuse all alcohol.
4. Decide not to worry about my calorie limit over the weekend—have a good weekend and get back on track after the weekend.
5. Take my cooler with low-calorie food so I can eat lightly during the day (e.g., fill up on fruit) and save up some calories to have a burger and a drink (work out calories before) in the early evening.
6. Take cooler, eat lightly and save calories for a burger, and take some low-calorie mixers as an alternative to alcohol.

Step 4: Think through the likely effectiveness and feasibility of each solution.
1. Decide not to go—probably not a good idea. I will be letting my friends down, as we planned this some time ago. I will feel fed up and lonely over the weekend, will miss all the fun, and may well overeat because I am so bored and fed up.
2. Eat nothing all day to save calories. This does not usually work. I will be so hungry by evening I may well exceed my calorie limit anyway. Also I will be irritable during the day and resentful that the others are eating, which may well spoil the weekend.
3. Take my own low-calorie food. This might be helpful, but I will still be tempted to have a burger and a drink and will be resentful that the others are doing so.
4. Decide not to worry about calorie limit. This may make the weekend easier and even more enjoyable in some ways, but I want to lose weight and I am sure I will regret not trying to stick to my limit. Also

it may be hard to get back on track once the weekend is over—I may start putting it off.

5. Take cooler and food for the day and save calories for burger and measured drink in evening. This could work. I might still find it difficult when others are having a cooked breakfast, but it will be easier than not eating at night.

6. Eat lightly from cooler, save calories for burger, have low-calorie mixers instead of alcohol. This might work. I prefer these to alcohol, but if they get warm they will be less pleasant. Also may be awkward not to drink at all and have my own supplies.

Step 5: Choose the best solution, or combination of solutions.
I will take some food with me in a cooler so that I will be able to eat lightly during the day and save some calories for a burger in the evening. I will also take some low-calorie mixers with me, and have some of these, but also allow myself to have a drink.

Step 6: Define the steps required to carry out the chosen solution and act on the solution.

1. The steps required: I need to plan exactly what to take in the cooler, so that I eat enough to ensure that I don't feel hungry, but also to make sure I have enough calories left over for a burger and a drink in the evenings. I need to work out how many calories there are likely to be in the burger and drinks, and I will calculate how many calories I will have left for the rest of the day. I will take plenty of salad and fruit with me, as I like these and they will help me not to feel hungry or deprived.

2. Acting on the solution: I took the cooler as planned, and this helped me resist the urge to eat "fast foods" most of the day; although I did give in on one day and ate some bacon on toast at breakfast time, as everyone else was having a cooked breakfast and it smelled wonderful.

Evaluating the problem-solving process.
I was fairly pleased with the problem-solving process. The extra bacon sandwich meant that I went over my calorie goal on one day, but I managed to stay under the calorie goal later in the week, bringing my average calories for the week close to the goal. I discovered that the cooler is heavy to carry around, which makes me reluctant to use it again. I plan to buy a lighter cooler before our next camping trip, and I will probably use a similar strategy again.

Addressing Limited Weight Loss

If the patient's weight is not decreasing at a reasonable rate (average loss of 1–2 lb or 0.5–1 kg per week), the therapist should review his or her compliance in detail. If the patient is clearly experiencing problems adhering to the 1,500-calorie limit, these should be directly addressed using a problem-solving approach. As always, patients should be encouraged to generate their own solutions.

If the patient appears to be adhering to the calorie goal but the therapist suspects the recording might be inaccurate, then the therapist should explain that the lack of weight loss is likely to be due to inaccuracy in the recording of energy intake or problems in calorie counting, or both, and that it is essential that the patient and therapist work together to find out exactly what the problem is. (It is of the utmost importance that this explanation is presented in a way that does not suggest that the therapist thinks the patient is lying.)

If the patient appears to be managing to adhere to the calorie limit, and the therapist does not suspect that the recording is inaccurate, then the patient and therapist should discuss the possibility of lowering the calorie goal to accelerate the rate of weight loss. If this seems appropriate, the therapist should suggest a 1,200-calorie limit, and then help the patient identify ways of cutting out the further 300 calories from his or her diet. Therapists should not introduce this new lower calorie limit unless they are reasonably confident that patients are going to be successful in adhering to it. (In some cases the therapist and patient may decide to move toward the 1,200-calorie limit in two steps; e.g., 1,350 then 1,200.) The patient's adherence to the new calorie limit will clearly be a focus of subsequent sessions. Problems adhering to the new limit should be addressed along the lines described above and in Chapter 5.

Determining When to Transfer to Weight Maintenance

As the patient's rate of weight loss begins to decline, therapists should begin to introduce the notion that it would be asking too much of the patient to maintain indefinitely his or her present level of food restriction. Doing this would be setting himself or herself up to fail as the research evidence indicates that people find it increasingly difficult to maintain dietary restraint after about 4 to 6 months, however successful they have been up to that point. Therapists should explain that a time will come when it will become clear that it would be best for the patient to stop trying to lose weight and instead start to learn how to maintain his or her new weight.

An issue of central importance to this treatment is deciding when the patient should stop attempting to lose further weight and instead move on to weight maintenance. Below are guidelines for deciding when to make this transition:

1. *When the rate of weight loss shows clear signs of slowing down despite good apparent compliance with energy restriction and calorie counting.* The research on the treatment of obesity suggests that the rate of weight loss decreases (with most treatments) by 6 months (Wadden et al., 1999; also see Wilson & Brownell, 2002). Although the explanation for this is not well understood, it is presumably due to the combination of waning compliance, decreased energy needs due to physiological changes, and a decrease in the en-

ergy expenditure associated with physical activity. Whatever the mechanism, it is observed as a progressive decline in the rate of weight loss. If this occurs despite apparent good compliance, then the therapist should begin to introduce the notion of "acceptance" (see Chapter 8), the goal being to help the patient realize that it is time to move on to weight maintenance.

2. *When the rate of weight loss shows clear signs of slowing down due to declining compliance with energy restriction.* In this case, therapists have two options: Either the decline in compliance can be addressed as a potentially soluble problem (see above), or it can be viewed as difficult to solve (perhaps due to patient burn out), and taken as an indication that it is time to move on to weight maintenance. The best policy is to be frank with the patient and discuss these two options, making it clear that continuing weight loss will become progressively more difficult given the three barriers noted earlier: difficulty maintaining continued dietary restraint; compensatory physiological changes, and decreased energy cost of physical activity.

If the patient and therapist conclude that compliance could be improved, then it is appropriate for this to be the immediate goal and the earlier guidelines should be followed. On the other hand, as treatment progresses beyond the half-way point (in our experience, beyond week 20), it becomes more appropriate to move on to weight maintenance. It is most important that this move is viewed as a positive and important next step rather than "resignation to an unhappy fate" (Wilson, 1996).

3. *About 3 months before the end of treatment.* At this point (which in the Oxford study was at week 30), the move over to weight maintenance should be made in order to allow sufficient time to practice the skills required (see Chapter 11). All patients should be forewarned of the need to make this transition, whatever their actual weight and ongoing rate of weight loss.

4. *Patients whose BMI reaches 22.* These patients should also move from weight loss to weight maintenance. They will also need to be forewarned of the need for this transition, the justification being that at a BMI of 22, their weight-related health risks will have been minimized and any further weight loss may do more harm than good (as well as being difficult to maintain). Once again, the transition should be viewed as a positive and important next step in long-term weight control.

CHAPTER 5

Module III: Adressing Barriers
to Weight Loss

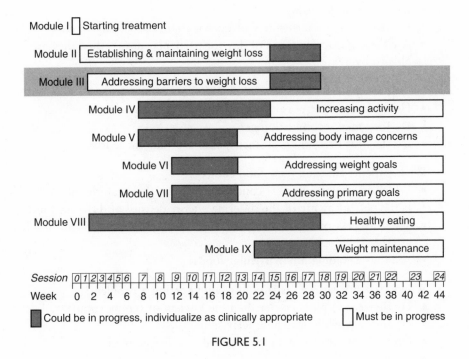

FIGURE 5.1

In the course of trying to lose weight, most patients will encounter a variety of obstacles. The goals for this module are as follows:

1. To identify behavioral and cognitive barriers to weight loss.
2. To help patients address these barriers as they arise.

Strategies for discerning obstacles and assisting patients in dealing with them are presented in detail below.

Identifying Barriers to Weight Loss

The identification of barriers to weight loss is achieved in two complementary ways: First, many can be identified by scrutiny of the patient's monitoring records, and, second, they can be sought more systematically using the "Barriers to Weight Loss Checklist" (see below).

Reviewing the Monitoring Records

When reviewing patients' monitoring records, therapists should look for potential barriers to weight loss. In doing so, the following points should be assessed:

- When patients eat (i.e., their temporal pattern of eating):
  - Do they eat formal meals (eating within the brackets)?
  - Do they snack or "pick" at food (eating outside the brackets)?
  - Are there any long periods with no eating?
  - Do they skip meals?
  - Is their eating pattern stable or does it change from day to day?
  - Are there particular times of day (or particular days) when they are liable to overeat?

- How much patients eat:
  - How big are their portion sizes?
  - Do they take second helpings?
  - Do they eat everything on their plate? Do they eat leftovers?

- What patients eat (i.e., their food choice):
  - Which foods (and drinks) contribute most to their calorie intake?
  - Is the patient aware of the differing energy density of different foods?
  - What aspects of their eating do they view as excessive (identified by asterisks)?
  - Are they avoiding any particular foods?

- Where patients eat (i.e., is stimulus-bound eating a problem?):
  - Do they eat in places other than the kitchen or dining room?
  - Do they eat while watching television?
  - Do they eat while driving or engaged in other activities?

- Other problems with eating:
  - Do they have discrete episodes of overeating?
  - Do they experience "loss of control" at the time (i.e., either a sense of being out of control, or not being able to resist eating, or not being able to stop eating once they have started)?

The therapist should consider all these issues. It is a matter of judgment whether to mention them at the time that they are identified or to delay highlighting them until later on. In general, if the patient is progressing well with reasonable behavioral compliance and resulting weight loss, then it is often best to delay addressing these issues until they become more relevant. This is likely to happen as patients' rate of weight loss invariably decreases over time. On the other hand, if these potential barriers actually appear to be limiting progress, then they should be highlighted and addressed.

Using the Barriers to Weight Loss Checklist

A complementary method for identifying potential barriers to weight loss involves using the "Barriers to Weight Loss Checklist" (see Table 5.1, next page; also reproduced as Handout K). This lists the most common obstacles to weight loss. It is designed to be completed by the patient and therapist together in part of a treatment session. Exactly when it is best completed varies from patient to patient. If progress is good, its completion is not a matter of urgency, although it should be completed if there are signs that the rate of weight loss is slowing, as this may be evidence of declining compliance. If progress is limited or erratic, the checklist should be completed early on as it may well highlight sources of difficulty that need to be addressed.

Addressing Barriers to Weight Loss

General Resistance to Treatment

Within a few weeks of starting treatment, it will be clear if there is resistance to change. This is likely to be expressed in one or more of the following ways:

- Failing to attend appointments
- Being late for appointments
- Repeatedly requesting to reschedule appointments
- Displaying an oppositional attitude in sessions (e.g., repeated challenging of the information provided or the necessity of performing homework assignments)
- Not complying well with homework assignments

The therapist should be on the alert for such signs of resistance. At first it is sufficient to take note of it (rather than raise the issue with the patient) while taking care to explain in detail the rationale for the treatment and its procedures and the need to complete the homework assignments. If this does not resolve matters, the problem will need to be directly addressed and the basis for the patient's resistance identified. The topic should be raised in a nonconfrontational manner. For patients to be able to speak freely, they should not have any sense that their comments will be taken as a criticism of the therapist.

Once the therapist has some idea of the nature of the patient's concerns, these should be addressed within the limits imposed by the weight problem and this form of treatment, as illustrated by the following vignette.

A patient was repeatedly late for sessions. She also frequently cancelled sessions at the last minute. The therapist was aware that there were a number of possible explanations for this behavior—such as the patient's generally chaotic approach to life, or that there could be a problem with motivation.

TABLE 5.1

Barriers to Weight Loss Checklist

Below is a list of commonly encountered barriers to weight loss. Please consider which (if any) apply to you, and place a tick in the relevant column.

	No	To some extent	Yes
Accuracy of recording:			
Is absolutely everything written down?			
Do you accurately measure your portions?			
Do you carefully calculate calories?			
Weighing and weekly reviews:			
Are you weighing yourself once a week?			
Are you holding weekly review sessions?			
Your eating pattern (i.e., when you eat):			
Do your eating habits vary greatly from day to day?			
Do you eat regular meals and snacks through the day?			
Do you skip any meals?			
Do you go for long periods without eating?			
Do you tend to nibble or pick at food?			
Are there particular times of day (or particular days) when you are liable to overeat?			
Do you have "binges" (large or small)?			
Your portion sizes:			
Are your portion sizes on the large side?			
Do you take second helpings?			
Do you always "clean your plate"?			
Do you eat leftovers?			
Your choice of foods and drink:			
Are you prone to eat energy-rich (i.e., high-fat) foods?			
Are you actively avoiding any foods?			
How you eat:			
Are you someone who eats very rapidly?			
Do you eat in places other than the kitchen or dining room?			
Do you eat while watching television?			
Do you eat while driving or engaged in other activities?			
Is your eating planned in advance?			
Do you eat directly from packets or containers?			
Other obstacles to weight loss:			
Have you lost your motivation to lose weight?			
Are you prone to stress-related eating?			
Are you liable to eat when bored?			
Does thinking in black-and-white terms undermine your attempts to lose weight?			
Are you facing other obstacles to losing weight?			

Initially the therapist decided to try a practical approach and assess her patient's response to this. She made an overt point of ending sessions on time regardless of how late the patient arrived to avoid reinforcing the patient's behavior. With regard to the cancellations, she raised the topic in this way: "Since you've had to rearrange a few sessions lately due to work commitments, I wonder if we should try to find a more convenient time to meet. We could have evening appointments, if you thought that might make it easier for you to get here."

In spite of these efforts, the patient continued to arrive late and cancel sessions. This was impeding progress in treatment. The therapist decided that the time had come to address the situation more directly. At the next session she said, "I've noticed that it seems difficult for you to get here sometimes, yet to get the most out of treatment it is really important that people attend regularly and for full sessions. For some people, not being able to get here is related to how they feel about the treatment—such as being unhappy about their rate of weight loss or not believing this type of treatment will work for them. Do you have any concerns of this type?"

The patient replied that she was eager to make the most of treatment, but that she was so busy it was hard for her to fit everything in. The therapist reminded her that the treatment could only be really effective if she made it a high priority in her life. The therapist suggested that they review the pros and cons of pursuing weight loss in order to make a thorough assessment of whether the patient wanted to make the commitment required. Following this review, the patient concluded that she really did want to continue with treatment. The therapist recommended that for homework the patient try problem solving to identify how she could protect time for attendance at sessions and for doing the necessary homework. The patient and therapist agreed that they would then review this plan thoroughly in the next session.

A similar approach may be taken with patients who repeatedly do not complete homework assignments. There is one significant additional factor to consider when homework is not completed: the therapist's behavior in relation to the homework. Therapists should ensure that they are following the principles outlined in Chapter 4 for assigning homework (see Table 4.2). It is particularly important that the rationale for homework assignments is clearly explained to the patient, that assignments are agreed upon collaboratively, that the tasks are manageable, and that the therapist reviews the homework in subsequent sessions. If patients are faced with assignments that they see as overwhelming or irrelevant, they are unlikely to devote much energy to them. Furthermore, if the patient does make an effort with homework but the therapist fails to devote attention to it, then the patient will be less motivated to complete future assignments.

A patient had been making somewhat halfhearted attempts at following the homework assignments and had been passive in treatment sessions. Her weight loss was modest. In session 4, the therapist raised her concerns about the patient's progress. The patient acknowledged that she was not happy with the treatment. She felt that it involved an inordinate amount of effort for little gain, whereas she had seen advertisements for treatments that produced much greater and faster weight loss. She had been considering ceasing to attend.

The therapist thanked her for being so open. She asked the patient for more details about the other treatments. It emerged that she was referring to treatments using very-low-calorie diets (VLCDs). The therapist explained that such treatments have been extensively studied, and that they do indeed produce fast and dramatic weight loss, but the weight lost is almost invariably regained even if great effort is put into post-VLCD weight maintenance (see Wadden & Berkowitz, 2002).

The therapist then spent time reviewing the rationale underlying the present treatment. The main points covered were as follows:

- The treatment addresses problems that may well account for the limited success of other treatments (i.e., it addresses barriers to successful weight maintenance), and it uses procedures that work in other areas (e.g., eating disorders, anxiety disorders).
- Many treatments produce faster and greater weight loss than this treatment, but the lost weight is almost always regained after the end of treatment.
- It is generally accepted that the priority in obesity treatment is to find a treatment that produces lasting weight loss. This treatment has this potential.
- It is essential to take a long-term perspective on weight problems and their treatment. Many clinics and treatments offer "quick fix" solutions, but they are not a long-term solution because the weight lost is regained. It is demoralizing for people to find that they have regained the weight that they had lost, and they tend to blame themselves rather than the inadequacy of the treatment provided.
- This treatment takes a long-term perspective and although the weight loss it produces may well be not as great (or as rapid) as the patient would like, the possibility that it will be enduring must always be kept in mind.

The patient said that she found it helpful reviewing these matters. She had lost sight of the positive features of the treatment. The therapist asked the patient to keep her informed about her concerns so that they could be openly discussed when they arose rather than remaining unspoken. The patient's compliance and attitude to treatment improved markedly from this point onward.

A minority of patients have difficulty in complying with the ongoing home-work assignment of recording their food and calorie intake.

Another patient was struggling to lose weight. She found calorie counting objectionable and felt very restricted by her calorie target. The therapist was in a difficult position because encouraging the patient to count calories accurately and stick to the target were important to ensure successful weight loss, but pushing too hard for this might have made this volatile patient angry, thus risking her withdrawing from treatment.

The following text is a verbatim record of some of the negative statements the patient made in a single session:

"... I am learning the calorie counting, but I find it difficult. I am hungry half the time, but I've usually already gone over my limit. If I ate what I really wanted I would be well over ...

"... and as for this business of no foods being restricted, well they are, because all food is high in calories. Only salad is not, and you cannot fill up on salad in this [cold] weather ...

"... if you have a sandwich, just two bits of bread and something between them, that's 400 calories gone already, and a 7-ounce baked potato sounds great, but it's only that big [gestures with hands to show very small potato] ...

"... low-fat foods are more expensive, and if I buy special stuff for me the rest of the family just eat it ...

"... my daughter keeps telling me I'll never lose weight like this. She says counting everything will make me think about food all the more ...

"... there was no way I was going to record over the weekend while my friends were visiting because I knew I would go over my calorie target, and I just was not prepared to sit and work it out ...

"... and I will not be able to do my diaries on Thursday and Friday, because I am going away to a funeral ..."

By taking care to acknowledge the patient's difficulties, highlighting her successes and setting modest goals, the therapist was able to make sure the patient left the session with a specific plan, and in the longer term helped her to lose a significant amount of weight. The therapist did this by being sympathetic ("Self-monitoring is difficult and a bit of a chore"), but firm ("Accurate monitoring is the key to this treatment working; without it, it's like tying your hands behind your back") about the need to continue with the self-monitoring.

In addressing this patient's problems with self-monitoring, the following strategies were helpful:

- Empathizing:

TH: It is true, calorie counting is a hassle—and it is hard work.

TH: It sounds like your daughter's comments were not helpful.

- Exploring issues while remaining nonjudgmental:

TH: What made you think that?

TH: Why might you not record when you go away for the funeral?

- Noting ambivalent statements and using them to move toward the desired goal:

P: This calorie counting thing, I just can't keep up with it. . . . On the other hand, if I go on vacation and don't stick to it, I will wish I had.

TH: So maybe it is helpful to think in the longer term. In the short term, calorie counting certainly does take time, and you do have to restrict your food. But if you look at it in the long term, the weight loss part is only for a certain period, then after you start maintenance, we will be thinking about stopping calorie counting, and there will be more flexibility in what you can eat.

- Highlighting positive achievements:

TH: What would you say you've accomplished this week?

TH: That is great, you weighed yourself at a time when it might have seemed easier not to; you started recording again right away after the weekend; and even when you were not recording, you still made some careful choices.

- Negotiating manageable goals:

TH: When you go away for the funeral, how about just noting the food down— not recording the calories—just to keep a track of things. Do you think that would be possible?

P: Well yes, but I don't think it will be accurate.

TH: No, but it might help just to keep a note—like you did the other day when you ate out. You did a great job then.

- Problem solving:

TH: Perhaps we could list some food that you like and that would help to fill you up?

TH: Perhaps we can devise a plan to stop your family from eating your special food?

- Correcting misunderstandings:

TH: You're right that food does have to be restricted while you are losing weight. What I was saying last time was that no food is "forbidden." So, if you really want to eat chocolate or pastry, for example, you can, but you do need to add up your calories for the day.

Some patients complain that counting calories makes them more preoccupied with what they are eating. In such cases the therapist can respond that this often does happen initially, and in fact it can be helpful, as it increases patients' awareness of what they are eating and so helps them to change.

In reviewing patients' concerns about treatment, therapists must keep patients aware of the inescapable fact that to lose weight, they will have to eat less than they used to eat; and that for successful long-term weight maintenance, they will have to adopt new eating habits and attitudes permanently.

When patients do not view their weight as a "problem," this is a particular obstacle to change. Although this is positive is some respects—in that it indicates that they have not been affected by the social pressures to be slim—it is not appropriate on health grounds. People with obesity are at increased risk of a variety of health problems, however fit or healthy they feel at present (see Chapter 3). This must be explained to them. They need to reduce their weight and adopt a healthy diet and active lifestyle if they are to reverse this increased risk of illness. In discussing these issues, it may be appropriate to adopt a short-term and long-term "pros and cons" approach, as outlined in Chapter 3.

A patient said during her initial appointment that she had never attempted to lose weight before, and that she was unsure how she felt about monitoring her food intake. She attended sessions 0–2, and completed daily monitoring sheets, although she did not provide many details on these, and the calorie calculations appeared inaccurate.

On week 3, the patient did not attend. The therapist phoned her, and the patient said that she had forgotten about her appointment. A suitable time for the following week was agreed, but when the appointment time came, the patient phoned to say that she was unable to attend. A new appointment was arranged for a week later.

When the patient arrived, she said she had forgotten to complete her monitoring records. She also reported that she had been busy and had not managed to buy a kitchen scale.

During the session, the therapist addressed the patient's motivation by asking her to list the pros and cons of complying with treatment. Below is a summary of the points that emerged:

Pros
- Health reasons—especially existing asthma and knee problems, which appear to be aggravated by weight. Also worries about risk of heart disease.
- Fitness—would like more energy (walking upstairs tired her out).
- Self-esteem and self-confidence—these had been adversely affected by comments about her weight from her partner and daughter.
- Sports—wanted to be able to go swimming again without embarrassment.

Cons

- Time pressure—had a hectic schedule as a student with a part-time job and a child. Difficult to make time to complete self-monitoring sheets (which took her longer than other patients as she was dyslexic).
- Interpersonal problems—the patient reported that she had severe relationship difficulties and was seriously considering ending her relationship with the partner she had lived with for 5 years. She felt unsure whether weight loss would be a "pro" or a "con" concerning any future relationship.

Each of the listed items was explored in detail, starting with the cons. The therapist then asked the patient to identify which items on the list appeared to be short-term ones and which were long-term. The patient was asked to take a copy of the list with her, and to consider the items and see if she could think of any more points of relevance before the next session.

At the end of the session, the patient said she realized there was never a "right time" to begin treatment, as there would always be other pressures, but she wanted to give the treatment a try. As she could not remember the reasons for self-monitoring, the therapist restated these. The patient stated that she had found it useful to self-monitor during the 2 weeks she had succeeded in monitoring, and she said she would begin self-monitoring again. She decided that, as she had tended to be forgetful, she would put notes on her lunch box and fridge to remind her to record her intake. She also identified a time in the coming week when she would be able to buy a kitchen scale.

After the session the therapist reflected that it would be important not to rush through material with this patient. Instead, she planned to progress through the treatment manual rather more slowly than she did with other patients.

Hunger

Hunger is to be expected on an energy-restricted diet. To help patients deal with hunger the following procedures should be tried:

- Explain that hunger is to be expected. It is a good sign, because it is evidence that they are successfully restricting their food intake.
- Help patients reduce their intake of energy-dense foods (see Chapter 4), because, as a result, a greater quantity of food can be eaten, thereby helping to minimize hunger.
- Encourage patients to eat at regular intervals through the day.
- Ensure that patients are not eating too little (i.e., not less than 1,200 calories daily).

- Suggest that they engage in distracting activities as hunger tends to wane over time.

Many patients are concerned because they feel extremely hungry when they start restricting their food intake. Clearly, this is to be expected, but it is rarely as bad as the patient predicts it will be. One patient who had a very high energy intake prior to commencing treatment found that she adapted quickly. After 3 weeks she reported:

> I am getting used to this. I am surprised I used to eat as much as I did. I had just got into the habit of thinking I needed that much food when actually this [1,500 kcal] is plenty. Some days I still go over; I eat too much food just because I like the look of it—I am still adjusting. I definitely do not need as much food as I thought I did. I really thought I would be feeling panicky all the time, looking at my plate and seeing measly portions and thinking that just will not be enough—but it is fine, I am surprised I had not worked this out before!

Accuracy of Recording

Some patients fail to record everything that they consume or to calculate their calorie intake accurately. This may not be deliberate, but nevertheless it can interfere with weight loss, as patients may be consuming far more energy than they think. Also, it can be demoralizing—patients may think that they are making an effort to restrict their energy intake and not seeing any results from their efforts. This may lead to the belief that, no matter what they do, they cannot control their weight, and eventually to the view that treatment is unlikely to be helpful. If this appears to be the case, the need for accurate recording must be stressed again. It is important that this is done in a nonjudgmental way so that it does not seem to patients that they are being accused of being untruthful. These points are illustrated by the following conversation between a patient (P) and her therapist (TH) below:

> P: I am really disappointed, I thought my weight might have gone down a bit today.
>
> TH: What did your scale at home say?
>
> P: Well, my weighing day is Friday. There was no change then, but I thought it might have come down a bit since then.
>
> TH: Looking at your graph, your weight loss has been a bit "on and off" over the last few weeks. How are you feeling about that?
>
> P: I really would like to lose some more weight, especially before I go on vacation.
>
> TH: It sounds frustrating for you. Your calorie intake looks fine though. Are you confident that you are recording everything? Is there anything that might be getting in the way of keeping truly accurate records?
>
> P: No, I don't think so, I definitely have not left anything out.

TH: Is there anything else you can think of that might have changed since you first started? Would it help if we got out some of your earlier diaries to compare them with your latest ones? We might be able to detect problems that might be interfering with your weight loss.

P: Well I've more or less already done that. I'm sticking to much the same pattern that I had when I started.

TH: OK, let's review matters. We know that if you stick to 1,500 calories a day and record accurately, then you must lose weight, and since that is not happening at the moment, we must be missing something. What some people have found helpful in this situation is to try a week of really meticulous recording. Think yourself back to your first week in treatment—when you weighed every single item, down to the last scrape of butter or the ounce of milk you put in your tea; when you wrote down each olive as you popped it in your mouth. Try repeating this level of accuracy for the next week. Some people find that after a while it is easy not to weigh, say, their cereal in the morning, because they think it's the same every day. But just a little change in portion size here and there can be enough to swing the balance away from weight loss. How does that sound—as an experiment—to be "super-accurate" for a week? At least then we could rule out this type of problem if it does not help, but I can think of a few people it worked very well for. What do you think?

One other possibility to consider is that the patient is deliberately not recording some things because he or she is ashamed of them—for example, he or she may be binge eating (see section below on binge eating). If the therapist thinks that this might be the case, then the issue should be addressed directly, and the patient should be asked if this is a problem.

Temporal Pattern of Eating

The therapist should pay attention to the patient's temporal pattern of eating. As explained in Chapter 4, it is best to follow a pattern of regular eating consisting of breakfast, lunch, possibly an afternoon snack, an evening meal, and an evening snack. Patients should distribute their calories across these meals and snacks by planning ahead and keeping a running calorie total, and they should be discouraged from eating between meals and snacks. Adherence to this pattern helps protect against "picking," informal snacking, and binge eating, and thereby helps control energy intake.

Skipping Meals or Snacks

Skipping meals or snacks is not a good idea. It increases the risk of subsequent overeating. Some patients have a longstanding habit of not eating breakfast. Such patients should be advised that eating breakfast can help prevent overeating later in the day. It is certainly essential if the avoidance of breakfast appears to lead to subsequent overeating. On the other hand, if no problems seem to arise from not eating breakfast, there is no need to insist upon it.

Similarly, the importance of an evening snack has been stressed (in Chapter 4). This particularly applies to those patients who tend to overeat after their evening meal either in the form of informal snacking or frank binge eating. If such overeating does not occur, then there may be no need for the patient to have an evening snack.

Eating between Meals and Snacks

Any tendency to eat outside meals and planned snacks makes it difficult to adhere to the calorie limit. There are three approaches to this problem, all of which may be relevant:

1. *Decrease the risk.* This can be achieved by:

- Helping the patient to choose meals and snacks that are nutritious and satisfying and to eat at regular intervals through the day. Evening meals and snacks may be especially important as patients are likely to have difficulties at this time.
- Encouraging the patient to remove environmental stimuli that appear to lead to between-meal eating; for instance,
  - remove stocks of high risk foods,
  - store such foods out of sight, and
  - avoid places where between-meal eating tends to occur.

A patient was prone to eat outside her planned meals and snacks when she was handling food. This was a problem as her job involved cooking. The therapist asked her to suggest possible ways of addressing this problem. She suggested eating chewing gum when cooking since this would prevent her from "picking." This proved successful, and the habit was broken over a couple of months. The patient then abandoned the routine use of chewing gum, although she kept a supply at hand for days when she felt most tempted to pick.

---

2. *"Urge surf."* Urges to eat between meals and snacks can often be successfully addressed by "response delay" as, if resisted, such urges decay over time rather than increase as many patients fear. Patients need to have this explained to them. The therapist should discuss how the patient can choose to engage in activities incompatible with eating until the urge to eat declines to a manageable level. These activities should be engaging rather than passive (e.g., exercising rather than reading) and pleasurable rather than aversive (e.g., talking to a friend on the telephone rather than catching up on household chores). They may include telephoning or visiting friends, taking some form of exercise, or having a bath or shower. Patients should be asked to think what form of activity might work best for them.

3. *Identify and address specific triggers of between-meal eating.* Common triggers are adverse moods such as boredom, anxiety, depression, and anger.

There are two aspects to overcoming the tendency to respond to adverse moods by eating.

- *Becoming adept at identifying (as early as possible) and solving the types of problem that trigger the adverse mood.* For example, triggers might include having nothing to do, pressure at work, having an argument with a friend or partner. This requires that the patient becomes skilled at formal problem solving (see Chapter 4).
- *Coping with the adverse mood itself without recourse to eating.* This requires helping patients to become better at recognizing, accepting, and coping with their adverse moods. With most patients the three steps below can be taught and practiced with relatively little difficulty.

  1. *Recognizing adverse moods.* Patients should be encouraged to monitor and observe their mood state. The goal is to become better at identifying moods in an objective way.
  2. *Tolerating adverse moods.* Patients should also be helped to accept and bear adverse moods especially if they cannot be moderated immediately (e.g., it is acceptable to be angry at times, being angry is part of normal human experience, and it is appropriate to feel and express anger in certain situations). They need to learn that amplification is not an inherent property of adverse moods—that is, the adverse mood does not escalate until it becomes unbearable; rather it is likely to decline. Therefore, it is possible to "mood surf" by delaying an immediate response to the mood. This will help patients avoid negative reactions to adverse moods, which do tend to prolong or escalate these states (e.g., becoming increasingly anxious about being anxious).
  3. *Dealing with adverse moods.* This involves helping patients identify and practice ways of coping with adverse mood states. They should list the pros and cons of dealing with the mood directly as opposed to using eating to deal with it, with the focus being on the long-term outcome. In general, two strategies may be employed to this end (usually in combination with "mood surfing"):
     - *Distraction.* Patients should actively engage in an activity, other than eating, that will distract them from their mood—for instance, taking a walk, having a shower, calling a friend, and so on.
     - *Improving the mood.* They should try to remove the negative mood by engaging in pleasurable mood-modulating activities (e.g., listen to music, have a warm bath, etc.).

Helping the patient acquire and develop these strategies will take a number of sessions with specific incremental homework tasks being set and reviewed.

One patient observed that she often overate when she felt low after a difficult day at work, even though she was not especially hungry. She compiled a list of relaxing and enjoyable activities, such as listening to music, doing some gardening, or simply exchanging the news of the day with her family. She tried using these activities in place of eating and found that they helped her to feel better. She felt better still when she realized she had resisted the urge to eat.

Binge Eating

A subgroup of those with obesity have recurrent episodes of binge eating, or episodes of uncontrolled overeating. Generally these binges are superimposed upon a general tendency to overeat rather than occurring against a background of extreme dietary restriction (as in the eating disorder bulimia nervosa). If the binges are sufficiently frequent, such patients are said to have binge eating disorder (see Chapter 2).

Binge eating is encouraged by:

- eating in response to adverse moods such as boredom, depression, anxiety, or anger. This mechanism is especially prominent in patients with obesity, although other mechanisms may also contribute.
- eating too little and too infrequently. This creates physiological and psychological deprivation, which in turn encourages overeating.
- attempting to obey numerous extreme dietary rules; having a perfectionist attitude to adherence to them; viewing the breaking of these rules in black-and-white terms; and having a tendency to abandon restricting food intake once a rule is broken.

The procedures needed to tackle binge eating have all been covered earlier in this chapter. They are as follows:

1. Addressing affective triggers of binge eating by:
   a. addressing the precipitating situation using problem solving;
   b. learning to recognize and accept adverse moods (including "mood surfing");
   c. practicing dealing with adverse moods.
2. Establishing a pattern of regular eating.
3. Progressively introducing avoided foods and in a similar fashion tackling other dietary rules.

The relevance of these procedures varies from patient to patient and depends upon the mechanisms underlying their binge eating.

At assessment a patient reported that she had been binge eating regularly over the past few months and that this was a source of distress to her. She said that once she started eating she was unable to stop. She felt guilty and ashamed about her binges, which she kept secret from her family and friends. The therapist asked the patient to commence the treatment as would any other patient, by recording her intake and working to an agreed calorie target. After several weeks, the therapist commented that the patient was not recording any episodes of binge eating on her monitoring sheets. The patient explained how pleased she felt that she had not binge eaten at all since the start of treatment. They examined the reasons for this, and concluded that making an effort to eat regularly and recording everything she was eating appeared to have eliminated the binge eating.

Another woman reported at the initial assessment that she had been a regular binge eater for more than 10 years. During the first 15 weeks of treatment, she managed to keep to a goal of around 1,500 kcal / day, and she lost 33.5 lb (15.2 kg). She sometimes ate 500–1,000 calories of ice cream at a time, but she said that she no longer experienced a loss of control during such episodes, as she was planning her food in advance and keeping to a calorie goal. The therapist encouraged her to try eating smaller amounts of ice cream, so that she could develop the habit of leaving some in the tub, but the patient was reluctant to try this.

At week 17, the patient reported that she had started binge eating again and had stopped self-monitoring—although until this point she had been meticulous in her monitoring. The therapist drew attention to the patient's "black-and-white" style of thinking, including her total abandonment of self-monitoring when she had gone over her calorie goal, and her tendency to eat either a whole tub of ice cream or none at all. The therapist explained that self-monitoring could help to reduce binge eating by helping the patient to be more aware of what she was eating. They discussed ways in which the patient had managed to avoid the urge to binge eat over the previous 15 weeks, by distracting herself. They highlighted the positive changes she had already made.

The patient agreed to try leaving some food on her plate or in the carton instead of eating complete packages of food. She also decided to try not to eat directly from packets; to eat more slowly; to distribute her eating more evenly over the day so that she did not feel hungry, and to choose a wider range of food. She mentioned that she had been feeling under stress due to financial difficulties. With encouragement she was able to identify more positive ways to deal with stress, and she used the problem-solving approach to identify strategies to deal with the difficulties. She put most of these strategies into practice, and only reported one further episode of binge eating over the remaining 27 weeks of treatment. As binge eating had been a long-standing problem and had resurfaced during treatment, the therapist helped her to identify ways of dealing with any future recurrences. The weight maintenance plan (see

Chapter 11) contained a detailed summary of strategies for preventing binge eating.

For further information on the cognitive-behavioral approach to the treatment of binge eating, see Fairburn, Marcus, and Wilson (1993) and Fairburn (1995).

Portion Sizes

Many people with obesity have a tendency to eat unduly large portions of food. This possibility should be raised with the patient (and especially with those who are losing little weight). They should be asked how their portion sizes would compare with those of others both inside and outside their family. (In some families everyone tends to eat large portions and therefore the patient may view a large portion as "average" in size). Of course, accurate calorie counting (and most especially the weighing of food) should detect the phenomenon, although it may be missed when patients eat out because, at such times, it may hard to quantify what is eaten.

If it appears that the patient may be eating unduly large portions, then this should become a focus of treatment. Patients should be helped to progressively reduce portion size either by decreasing the amount on their plate or by practicing leaving food. Their success should be assessed at subsequent sessions. One strategy that can be helpful is to suggest that patients eat off smaller plates for a while.

The energy density of food may also be relevant here (see Chapter 4). Some patients feel that they are not eating enough food once they restrict their portion size. A solution to this problem is for them to change to foods that are less energy-dense (generally lower-fat foods) because this allows a greater quantity of food to be eaten.

Food Choice

In the weight loss phase of this treatment, patients' food choice is not a major focus so long as their diet is not unduly unhealthy and they are succeeding in losing weight. To avoid overburdening patients with behavioral demands, they should be advised to do just two things (see Chapter 4): eat a broad range of foods and reduce their consumption of energy-dense food (i.e., high-fat food). On the other hand, in the long-term establishing a healthy diet is a priority. This subject is addressed in Chapter 10.

Certain problems relating to food choice may be encountered during weight loss:

1. *Some patients eat an extremely poor diet from a nutritional standpoint.* For example, they may not be eating a major food group (e.g., fruit) or nutrient (e.g., calcium). Under such circumstances, therapists must point out the nu-

tritional consequences of such a diet and help patients incorporate the missing items. Therapists need only look for obvious deficiencies. For comprehensive nutritional information, see Garrow, James, and Ralph (2000) and Ziegler and Filer (1996).

2. *Some patients are used to eating a high-fat diet, and their attempts at dietary restriction simply involve eating smaller amounts of these foods rather than simultaneously increasing their intake of other foods.* This is a problem because, usually, patients cannot sustain such restriction over time and any increase in the quantity of food eaten results in a disproportionately large increase in the calories consumed. This is likely to be a particular problem for long-term weight maintenance. These patients need to be helped to decrease their intake of high-fat foods while increasing their intake of less energy-dense alternatives. Guidelines for doing this are provided in Chapter 10. If there is a significant problem relating to food choice, these guidelines should be introduced at this point in treatment.

A patient had a strong preference for high-fat foods. She managed to lose weight successfully, but was reluctant to alter her food choice. In order to lose weight, she chose to simply cut back on the amount of high-fat food that she ate, rather than to make significant changes to her eating habits. The therapist encouraged her to consider low-calorie alternatives and to increase her intake of fruits and vegetables. The patient did make one or two attempts to experiment with foods outside her preferred range, but she was unwilling to persevere along these lines. She rejected alternative foods if they were in any way disadvantageous to her (e.g., she refused to eat certain vegetables on the grounds that cooking them made her apartment smell).

The patient managed to lose 24.5 lb (11.1 kg) by reducing her calorie intake, but her reluctance to modify her food choice created a major barrier to weight maintenance, as even a small increase in the quantity of food that she was eating resulted in a disproportionately large increase in her caloric intake.

Food Avoidance

Some patients adopt (or already have) a highly restricted diet in which they attempt to eat a narrow range of foods. Often these patients have a "black-and-white" style of thinking (known as dichotomous thinking), expressed in the form of rigid and brittle dietary rules and a tendency to overeat in response to any perceived breaking of these rules. They may talk about "good foods" (low-calorie foods) and "bad foods" (high-calorie foods), and they may try to completely avoid the "bad foods." These patients need to be encouraged to broaden their food choice by progressively introducing the avoided items into their diet. They should be taught that no food is "banned," and that it is better to allow oneself to eat small amounts of food which one likes, rather than to try never to eat the desired food. This is because banning a food that one likes often leads to cravings for this specific food, and to excessive eating when one "gives in" to the desire to eat it.

Often the focus needs to be on the type of food avoided (e.g., chocolate) rather than on eating a particular amount of it. The goal is to help patients break the dietary rule that is restricting their eating, without triggering an episode of overeating. Specific homework tasks should be discussed. For example, the patient might plan to eat half a bar of chocolate during their morning break one day in the week, and throw the other half away immediately. The patient should be asked to predict what they think will happen (in terms of their behavior, thoughts, and feelings) with the therapist taking care to identify their specific fears. The patient should then be encouraged to try eating the food as planned, as a behavioral experiment, and to write down what happens. At the following session, the experiment should be discussed, and predictions should be compared with what actually happened (in terms of behaviors, thoughts, and feelings, and other relevant consequences—e.g., finding that eating one bar of chocolate does not cause significant weight gain or lead to binge eating).

When assigning the homework, it is important to discuss ways of preventing subsequent overeating following the consumption of the avoided food item. Patients might be encouraged to:

- not introduce the avoided food on a day on which they do not feel reasonably in control of their eating;
- be aware of the likely urge to overeat following consumption of the avoided food and to identify and counter the accompanying thoughts;
- engage in distracting activities afterward until the urge to overeat has waned to a manageable level.

This introduction of avoided foods needs to be practiced regularly until the patient's consumption no longer triggers fears of weight gain and urges to overeat.

A patient believed that while she was losing weight she must completely avoid chocolate. Prior to starting the treatment she had eaten several bars a day, in a habitual manner. She believed that once she started eating chocolate she would not be able to control her consumption of it, therefore it was best avoided. The therapist encouraged her to experiment with eating moderate amounts of chocolate in a planned fashion. The patient selected a suitable day, bought one single bar of chocolate, and planned a time when she would eat it. She found that she was able to enjoy the chocolate and did not crave more. From that point on, she began to include small amounts of chocolate into her calorie allowance from time to time.

Another patient liked chocolate cake but struggled to include it within her calorie goal because when she ate it she tended to eat large amounts, finding herself unable to stop at a "normal" portion. The patient found this distressing and felt that she could not control her intake of chocolate cake. She had perfectionist standards for her eating and a black-and-white thinking style, so that once she had overeaten she felt she had failed and became very miserable. This put her at risk for further overeating. The therapist encouraged her to try eating planned, measured amounts of chocolate cake. However, this was not wholly successful as she sometimes ate more than she had planned, and even if she did stop at the planned portion she felt unsatisfied.

Over her summer vacation, the patient decided to allow herself a slightly higher calorie goal. The therapist suggested this might be a good opportunity for her to experiment with her consumption of chocolate cake. The patient and the therapist discussed the problem, which they summarized as follows: Chocolate cake is desirable, but it is also high in calories. The patient wished to eat as much of it as she wanted, but as she knew that it was high in calories she felt she must consume as little as possible. However, when she consumed a small amount, she felt cheated and dissatisfied. She sometimes responded to this feeling by eating more and more until doing so was no longer pleasurable, by which time she felt guilty and a failure. Even if she did not eat more cake, she continued to feel cheated as she had not eaten as much as she wanted.

The patient actually did not know how much chocolate cake would constitute "as much as she wanted" because she had always tried to restrict her intake. She anticipated that it would be an unreasonably large amount and therefore felt doomed to restrict her intake; that is, she felt deprived before she had even started eating.

The therapist and patient agreed on an experiment. The patient would cut off a piece of cake that looked to her as if it would be satisfying, with no restriction on size or consideration of its calorie content. She would eat it and see how she felt. If she was not satisfied, she could eat more. When she felt satisfied, she would calculate (by assessing what remained of the cake) how many calories her portion contained.

The patient did this—and felt satisfied after the first piece she cut. Once she had calculated the calories consumed, she was delighted to discover that her "optimum" portion corresponded fairly closely to an "average" portion. After this she was able to eat moderate amounts of cake much more comfortably.

Style of Eating

The therapist should consider how patients eat. As explained in Chapter 4, it is best for eating to be planned and for meals to be eaten in a set place. Patients should savor their food rather than eat it automatically. The following points should be assessed as they apply to their eating in general and to episodes of overeating:

- *Speed of eating.* Food that is eaten quickly tends not to be noticed and therefore to be less satisfying. Patients who tend to eat rapidly should be encouraged to savor their food instead. Putting cutlery down between mouthfuls is one technique that helps people slow down their eating.

A patient who was a single parent found that she was eating her food rapidly so that she could be ready to clear away her children's plates as soon as they had finished eating. Another woman noticed that eating for her was simply a case of refueling when the opportunity arose. She did not notice the taste or texture of foods; indeed, sometimes she ate strange combinations of foods simply because they were the most readily available. In both cases the therapist encouraged the patients to eat "mindfully"; to take time to savor each mouthful and to notice tastes and textures.

- *Eating accompanied by other activities.* Performing other activities such as reading or watching television while eating is generally not a good idea because it may lead to overconsumption (as people are not aware of how much they have eaten when their attention is elsewhere). Instead patients should concentrate on what they are eating and enjoy it.
- *Place.* Formalizing eating by sitting down in a set place (rather than eating in a variety of places) encourages controlled eating.
- *Planning.* This should be encouraged as it reduces the risk of eating between meals. It is useful for patients to note the plan for the day at the top of the monitoring record.

Treatment was progressing reasonably well, but the patient had a tendency to exceed her calorie goal on occasions through lack of planning. Although she understood the importance of planning ahead, she was reluctant to do this on a day-to-day basis because she felt she would become obsessed with calories.

After a few weeks, the patient worked out a system that prevented her from exceeding her calorie goal but did not interfere with her desire for spontaneity and flexibility. This involved shopping twice a week and buying enough food (including several prepared dishes) to serve for the next 3 days. By doing this, she made sure that all the food that she had readily available was appropriate to her calorie goal, was quick and easy to prepare, and comprised things she liked. This allowed her to be flexible and, to a degree, spontaneous.

• *Eating directly from packages.* This tends to encourages overconsumption. Instead, patients should set out the food that they are going to eat and, before starting, put away the remainder.

Alcohol

For some patients, alcohol intake worsens their weight problem or interferes with treatment. Several mechanisms may be operating:

• Alcohol consumption may make a significant contribution to calorie intake.
• Alcohol may diminish the ability to exert dietary restraint (and some patients report that they feel more hungry after drinking alcohol).
• The environment in which alcohol is consumed may undermine dietary adherence. For example, snacks (e.g., nuts or chips) or other high-fat food may be available, and there may be social pressure to eat "fast food."

Therapists need to identify which of these obstacles is operating and tailor their advice accordingly. It is important to adopt a noncensorious attitude to the patient's drinking, and it may not be realistic to expect them to change long-established social habits. On the other hand, if the patient's drinking is proving an obstacle to weight loss, this needs to be discussed in detail and solutions sought using the problem-solving approach (see Chapter 4). For example, patients may decide to try to cut down the amount drunk on each occasion (e.g., by filling up on water first, thereby ensuring that they are not thirsty when they start to drink; and alternating alcoholic drinks with nonalcoholic diet drinks), or to decrease the number of times they drink in a week, or both. Some patients choose to totally revise their drinking habits and make a "fresh start."

Dietary Guidelines versus Dietary Rules

The therapist should be on the alert for cognitive processes that might impair adherence to the 1,500-calorie diet. A particularly common problem is the translation of dietary guidelines into inflexible rules. One example of this is translating the recommendation of reducing calorie intake into "I should never eat snacks or high fat foods." Another is seen in the way some patients become distressed or feel they have failed if they occasionally exceed the calorie goal even by small amounts. Patients should be reminded that the 1,500-calorie limit is a guideline for average calorie intake—it is not a rigid prescription. A goal is something to aim at, but patients are not expected to meet the goal every day. They might eat a bit more on some days and a bit less on other days, but they should aim for an average intake over the week of 1,500 calories per day.

For a few people, transforming dietary guidelines into rules is helpful. The lack of ambiguity helps their adherence. Unfortunately, for most people such rigid rules cause problems, both because they are inflexible and so are likely to be broken on occasion and because the usual reaction to breaking such rules is the temporary abandonment of attempts to restrict eating (as described earlier).

Often simply identifying "black-and-white" thinking, discussing its consequences and helping patients see how they could be less extreme without any detrimental effect, is enough to moderate this tendency, especially if they use their monitoring records to identify it in operation. Relevant homework may also be useful (typically including the planned breaking of a dietary rule). (Chapter 7 discusses black-and-white thinking in relation to body image problems.)

A patient felt strongly that she must achieve a calorie intake of less than 1,500 calories every day. If her daily intake was above this she felt she had failed, became downhearted, and was prone to give up. The therapist asked the patient why she felt it was so important that her calorie intake *must* be below 1,500 every day even though she had been told to average *around* 1,500 calories per day. The patient explained that in part it was related to her belief that if she did not lose weight, she would gain weight, and that she feared that exceeding 1,500 calories would precipitate weight gain. She also described how failing to stick exactly to her calorie goal indicated to her that she had lost control.

The therapist helped the patient to review the evidence for both of these beliefs. The patient monitored her weight change over several weeks and found that she continued to lose weight even when her average calorie intake was slightly greater than 1,500 calories per day. They also noted that although her calorie intake was strongly related to her weight loss, the relationship was not precise. The patient was able to see that as long as she stuck to *around* 1,500 calories per day, she lost weight, and that it was pointless to be too rigid about her calorie goal because other factors that affected her weight were beyond her control (such as her menstrual cycle). The therapist also prompted her to identify any evidence to suggest she was in control of her food intake—and she found plenty. The patient started to appreciate that keeping records, planning ahead for special occasions, losing weight, and reducing her intake of high-fat foods were all evidence of her ability to control her food intake. Her single measure of control (sticking to under 1,500 calories daily) had not been a good index of her ability to control her food intake.

Other Cognitive Barriers to Weight Loss

Other cognitive processes that appear to be barriers to weight loss may need to be addressed. For example, some patients have unrealistic goals regarding their rate for weight loss, and they become distressed if they do not lose a specific (and unreasonable) amount of weight during a given time period. They may then become discouraged and tempted to give up. One patient said:

> My father is really eager for me to have targets. He thinks you have got to have a goal to achieve anything. For me specific goals are the worst thing. I have goals I am working toward, but they do not hinge on a specific number so I cannot fail at them. If I am on the road toward my overall aim, it does not matter where I am along that road—just as long as I am still on it.

Patients need to be helped to adopt this attitude, with rigid, demanding goals being replaced by flexible and realistic objectives. The related and central topic of target weights is addressed in detail in Chapter 8.

Use of Food as a "Treat"

The use of food as a comfort, reward, or "treat" presents a particular obstacle to change. This use of food is generally longstanding, and it can undermine dietary compliance. To tackle this problem, the therapist must first identify it as such. Then the link between "self-nurturance" (i.e., addressing one's needs) and eating needs to be broken. The following strategy may be used:

1. *Review with patients whether eating does in fact make them feel better.* If it does, does the improvement last? Is it a good solution if one takes a long-term perspective?

2. *Patients should then be asked to practice breaking the link.* For example, the next time they have the urge to comfort or reward themselves with food, they should try delaying doing so for 15 minutes. This plan can be set up as an experiment to see whether the delay results in an increased need for the food or whether the urge to eat declines (as is almost invariably the case). In this way the patient learns that such urges do not have to be satisfied.

3. *Patients should be helped to identify and use other ways of comforting and rewarding themselves at these times.* Identifying good ways of rewarding themselves can be set as a homework task. They can then be used the next time the opportunity arises.

A patient decided to try "urge surfing" to help her cope with cravings to eat chocolate. The therapist suggested that she try using distracting activities while she was waiting for the urge to dissipate. In order to work out what kind of distracting activities might help, the therapist asked the patient to describe exactly what it was about the experience of eating chocolate that she liked so much. The patient described how she sat down with a cup of tea and some chocolate, and exactly how the chocolate felt in her mouth as the warm tea dissolved it. It appeared that there were several elements to the experience: a chance to sit down and relax; a sense of luxury; and the specific textures and tastes that the combination of tea and chocolate gave. The therapist and patient then considered alternative activities that might have some or all of these properties. The patient thought that sitting down, still with a cup of tea, stroking the cat, and enjoying the feeling of its soft fur might be one possibility. Other possibilities included having a candle-lit bath, and listening to a favorite piece of music.

Two other patients also ate for reasons other than hunger. One woman discovered that she was eating as a way of creating some time for herself—sitting down to eat was a pleasurable thing to do, which gave her a little time away from the seemingly unending tasks of being a working mother. This patient agreed to try other enjoyable and absorbing non-food related activities, such as needlepoint or word-search puzzles, and to work on being more assertive about making time for herself. Another patient ate while watching television after her husband and daughter had gone to bed. She found that having unstructured time (which she felt she should use for doing chores) triggered her to eat. In this case she was able to "reward" herself for spending part of this time doing chores by allowing herself to sit down and watch television for a while, perhaps with a glass of wine, but without food.

CHAPTER 6

Module IV: Increasing Activity

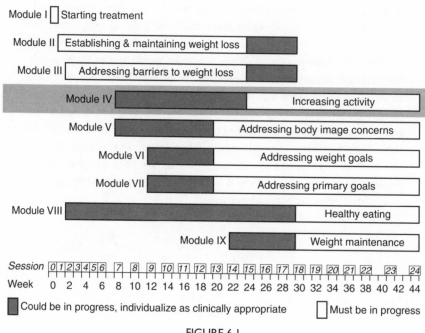

Module I ☐ Starting treatment

Module II Establishing & maintaining weight loss

Module III Addressing barriers to weight loss

Module IV Increasing activity

Module V Addressing body image concerns

Module VI Addressing weight goals

Module VII Addressing primary goals

Module VIII Healthy eating

Module IX Weight maintenance

Session 0 1 2 3 4 5 6 7 8 9 10 11 12 13 14 15 16 17 18 19 20 21 22 23 24
Week   0 2 4 6 8 10 12 14 16 18 20 22 24 26 28 30 32 34 36 38 40 42 44

☐ Could be in progress, individualize as clinically appropriate   ☐ Must be in progress

FIGURE 6.1

This cognitive-behavioral approach to the treatment of obesity does not place as much emphasis on exercise as many other treatments do. However, the treatment does view it as important to encourage patients to lead an active life, especially from the perspectives of successful weight maintenance and enhanced physical health.

The treatment draws a distinction between overall activity (and the lack of it in the form of sedentariness) and formal exercise (see below). Both can be addressed at the same time, but the emphasis of the treatment is primarily on increasing overall activity levels as those who adopt an active lifestyle are most successful at controlling their weight in the long term. Increases in formal exercising are welcomed but they are not a goal of treatment per se.

The goals of this module are the following:

1. To help patients increase overall activity levels.
2. To encourage adoption of formal exercise, if appropriate.

Determining When to Enter Module IV

The topics of activity and exercise are not raised in the early stages of treatment, because they are not viewed as essential for weight loss (see Figure 6.1). Instead, they are addressed at either of the following two points in treatment:

1. *If weight loss has been established, and the subject of activity or exercise is raised by the patient.* For example, some patients want to integrate increasing activity with dietary restriction. This is to be encouraged so long as it does not interfere with dietary compliance. In general it is best to do this informally rather than by entering this module (which should be delayed until later on). Therapists should portray such an increase in activity as a good means of enhancing health rather than as a supplementary means of weight control. Suitable activities should be identified and monitored as described below, and appropriate homework targets set. Patients should be reinforced for all progress that they make.

2. If not discussed already, we recommend that the subject of activity always be raised by around the middle of treatment (in our case it is always raised by week 24), as those who have an active lifestyle are most successful at controlling their weight in the long term. Clearly it is essential that this module be entered sufficiently early for patients to firmly establish a more active lifestyle before treatment ends.

The treatment uses a graded approach to increasing activity levels which may be divided into six steps. Steps 1–3 can be done in the same session. They involve education and the introduction of self-monitoring. In step 4 the findings of the self-monitoring are evaluated and, if indicated, in step 5 ways of increasing activity levels are introduced. An incremental approach is taken, with homework being assigned in each session and then progressively built upon. Step 6 addresses the long-term maintenance of activity levels.

Although not a goal of this treatment, any increase in formal exercise is encouraged. Means of facilitating formal exercise are described at the end of the module.

Increasing Overall Activity

Step 1: Distinguish the Three Forms of Activity

The therapist should explain to the patient that it is useful to distinguish three forms of activity:

1. *Being sedentary* (strictly speaking, a form of inactivity). This refers to sitting or lying down (e.g., watching television; being at a desk at work, resting in bed).
2. *Lifestyle activity.* This refers to incidental activity that is part of day-to-day life. It includes walking, standing, climbing stairs, household chores, light gardening, ordinary cycling, and gentle swimming.
3. *Formal exercise.* This is what people generally think of as exercise. To be classed as "formal exercise" in this context, it should involve exertion to the point that the pulse and respiratory rate are increased. It includes jogging, moderate-to-fast swimming, brisk walking or power walking, and fast cycling.

It should also be explained that there is evidence that people with obesity tend to be unusually inactive. This compounds the health risks associated with obesity (see Blair & Holder, 2002) and means that energy intake has to be lower than it might be otherwise.

Step 2: Explain the Benefits of Increasing Overall Activity and Correct Misconceptions about Exercise

There are three main reasons to increase activity levels:

1. To improve long-term weight maintenance. There is reasonably convincing clinical and research evidence that people who are more active are better at maintaining their weight in the long term (Blair & Holder, 2002). The basis for this is uncertain, but it is not thought to be simply an index of better compliance with other aspects of weight maintenance.
2. To reduce the health risks associated with obesity.
3. To increase calorie consumption. This is a modest effect. Patients must be told that increasing activity is not, even remotely, a substitute for dietary control. For example, in order to lose weight at a rate of around 1 lb (0.5 kg) per week it is necessary to create a daily energy deficit of some 500 calories. To achieve this by an increase in energy expenditure alone, it would be necessary for a 176-lb (79.8-kg) person to walk for 110 minutes per day, or cycle for 80 minutes per day, or swim (breaststroke) for 45 minutes per day in addition to their baseline level of activity.

Some people obtain other benefits from activity, including:

- feeling physically healthier;
- feeling better about themselves in general;
- having more social contact; and
- improving mood.

The therapist should check whether the patient believes any of the following common misconceptions about the relationship between physical activity and weight, and, if so, correct information should be provided.

1. *Exercise is of little value in weight control.* Modest amounts of regular exercise are thought to be important in helping prevent weight regain (see Wing & Klem, 2002).

2. *Only strenuous exercise will produce significant health benefits.*

a. It is generally agreed that building up to a total of 30 minutes per day of moderate-intensity activity on most days of the week confers significant health benefits (Blair & Holder, 2002). Moderate-intensity activities are those that make the person breathe harder and feel warmer—brisk walking is a good example.

b. Strenuous exercise results in a high calorie expenditure on a per-minute basis, but "lifestyle" activities may be easier to fit into a daily routine and sustain over the longer term. Therefore they can make a significant contribution to energy expenditure. For example, a 20-minute swim would result in an additional (i.e., above baseline activity level) calorie expenditure of 210 calories, but an hour's light gardening would use an extra 250 kcal, and may be fitted into the day in shorter blocks of time if this were more convenient. Another example might be weekly attendance at an aerobics class versus a daily 10-minute walk: each would achieve the same total additional calorie expenditure.

3. *Exercise leads to an increase in appetite.* Moderate exercise does not increase appetite and may in fact reduce it (Blundell, 2002). Furthermore, exercise helps people feel good about themselves and helps them avoid overeating in response to stress. (In addition, exercise is generally incompatible with eating, and so tends to be associated with eating less).

Step 3: Start to Monitor Activity Levels

As a first step in increasing activity level, the three forms of activity should be monitored. The therapist should therefore ask patients to start recording them in an "activity box" (see Table 6.1) on the back of the day's monitoring record (midnight to midnight).

> *Inactivity (sedentariness).* At the end of each day, the patient records the number of hours spent sitting or lying. For those patients who sit down at work, it may be best if they keep a running total in column 6 of their monitoring records.

TABLE 6.1

Box for the Daily Recording of the Three Types of Activity

Inactivity (hours)	
Lifestyle activity (steps)	
Formal exercise (minutes and type)	

Lifestyle activity. This may be quantified using a simple digital pedometer (which counts the number of steps taken during a day). These are readily available and inexpensive. It is our practice to lend one to patients. They should be asked to wear the pedometer each day for 2 weeks, and given instructions on its use.

Formal exercise. At the end of each day, the patient should also record in the activity box the number of minutes engaged in formal exercise (as defined above) and the type of exercise taken.

The handout "Monitoring Your Level of Activity" (Table 6.2; Handout L) summarizes these points and provides patients with details about how to record their activity level. The therapist should go through this handout with the patient.

Step 4: Evaluation of Activity Levels

In the next session, the therapist should assess the patient's monitoring of activity levels. Any difficulties should be identified and addressed. If the activity monitoring has been satisfactory, the therapist and patient should then together evaluate the findings.

Inactivity (sedentariness). The number of hours spent being inactive should be reviewed, noting any difference between weekdays and weekends.

Lifestyle activity. The patient's average step count should be assessed, once again noting any difference between weekdays and weekends. From our experience in the United Kingdom (using the Yamax Digi-walker SW-200), we offer the following suggested reference values:

Activity level	Steps per day
Very low	< 3,000 steps
Low	3,000–5,000 steps
Moderate	5,000–7,000 steps
High	> 7,000 steps

Formal exercise. Many people with obesity take no formal exercise (as defined above). The patient's baseline level of formal exercising should be noted. Although increasing its level is not a goal of this treatment, it is worth evaluating the patient's attitude to formal exercising with the goal of identifying one or more forms of exercise that the patient might be willing to consider starting (or increasing) at some point. If the patient is already considering increasing his or her level of formal exercise, this should be encouraged.

Step 5: Decreasing Sedentariness and Increasing Lifestyle Activity

Decreasing sedentariness and increasing lifestyle activity are best addressed at the same time.

TABLE 6.2

Information for Patients on How to Monitor Their Activity

MONITORING YOUR LEVEL OF ACTIVITY

The first step in increasing your level of physical activity is to measure how active you are now. To do this you need to measure the three forms of activity discussed in treatment.

Inactivity

At the end of each day recall as accurately as you can how many hours you have spent sitting or lying down. Do this for a 24-hour period (midnight to midnight) projecting forward for the few hours remaining in the day. Then record the number in an "activity box" drawn on the back of the day's monitoring record (see below). If you sit down at work, it may be best to keep a running total of the time spent sitting in column 6 of your monitoring record.

Lifestyle Activity

This term refers to incidental physical activities that are part of day-to-day life. It includes walking, standing, climbing stairs, household chores, light gardening, ordinary cycling, and gentle swimming.

With the exception of cycling and swimming, we recommend quantifying these activities in an approximate way (in terms of the number of steps taken) using a pedometer.

If you have a pedometer, you should wear the pedometer at all times except when in bed and engaging in formal exercise (see below). You should put it on first thing in the morning. To remember to do this, attach it to something you use first thing in the morning (e.g., a comb or hair brush) and return the reading to zero by pressing the reset button. Attach the pedometer to a belt or article of clothing at the side of your hips. Then, last thing at night, note the number of steps recorded in the day's activity box. Please note that you should ignore any calorie table that may come with the pedometer as such figures are generally misleading.

Formal Exercise

At the end of each day you should also record in the activity box the number of minutes spent engaged in formal exercise. To be classed as formal exercise, the exercise should involve exertion to the point that your pulse and breathing rate are increased. Such exercise includes jogging, moderate-to-fast swimming, brisk walking, and fast cycling.

Activity Box

The activity box summarizes your level of activity over the previous 24 hours. It should be drawn on the back of the day's monitoring record and completed at the end of the day. It should look like this:

Inactivity (hours)	8 hours in bed, 3 hours sitting
Lifestyle activity (steps)	3,860 steps
Formal exercise (minutes and type)	None today

Decreasing Sedentariness

If the patient is highly sedentary, the therapist and patient should review ways of tackling this problem. These can include reducing the amount of time spent sitting down watching television (by engaging in lifestyle activities such as going for walks or gardening) and sitting down less at work. In almost every case, watching less television is a simple and worthwhile goal. Specific incremental targets should be set and reviewed at subsequent sessions.

Increasing Lifestyle Activity

If the patient's step count indicates that he or she has a low (or very low) baseline level of lifestyle activity, a plan should be devised for increasing it. This is best done by asking patients how they think their level of lifestyle activity might be increased. The goal should be that they move up to moderate or high levels of activity (as defined above). They should be encouraged to look out for opportunities to be active. Choosing to involve someone else can be helpful. It can aid motivation (as both people can encourage each other), and it provides social contact. Possible forms of activity include the following:

- Standing up instead of sitting (e.g., when on the phone)
- Getting up to change the television channel instead of using the remote control
- Going for a (brisk) walk at lunchtime or in the evening
- Using the car less
- Getting off the bus or subway a few stops earlier
- Parking at the far side of parking lots

The use of stairs deserves special mention because it is a particularly good form of lifestyle activity. Patients should be encouraged to use stairs whenever possible (by making extra journeys and by minimizing their use of elevators and escalators). It may be appropriate to monitor the number of flights climbed per day.

Again, specific incremental targets should be set and reviewed at subsequent sessions. Going for a walk every day is a simple and worthwhile goal. Taking up an active recreation should also be encouraged. It is best if this activity is not exclusively seasonal as patients tend not to identify alternative activities for off-season periods. Also, there is a risk that the activities will not be restarted when the season resumes. The therapist should ask patients to consider how they will maintain an increase in activity in the long term. If appropriate, they should also be asked to consider how they will cope with seasons when it is not possible (or easy) to engage in their chosen activity, and the risk of not resuming the activity should also be discussed.

It is often worthwhile asking the patient to use the pedometer for a second 2-week period 4–6 weeks later to assess whether there has been any increase in activity.

After recording her activity level over a 2-week period, one patient noted that she spent many hours sitting down (her work was sedentary, and one of her main leisure activities was watching television). She also noted that she did no formal exercise. The patient stated that she was not eager to reduce the time she spent watching television, as it was the only time she had together with her husband, and also because she wanted to keep the evenings "chore-free." The therapist agreed that it was vital that the patient plan physical activity in a way that she felt did not impinge unduly on her time, and that she would not end up resenting. So, although the therapist might ideally have encouraged the patient to consider the possibility of less sedentary leisure activities, initially he decided to accept the patient's preference and look for other parts of her day where she could increase her activity level.

The patient thought over her options and decided that she would try to walk during her lunch hour at work. To help encourage herself and see the walks as purposeful, she decided to try walking to the post office to drop off the mail that she would otherwise take in her car at the end of the day. She decided to try this twice per week initially, in order to prevent the task seeming daunting. She also decided to enquire about the availability of yoga classes in her area as this was an activity she felt she would enjoy, and which she could do at the weekend when she had more free time.

Another woman who had previously been fairly sedentary decided to make walking her main activity. She gradually increased her walking, so that eventually she was walking to and from work, at lunchtime, and to the newstand when previously she would have used the car. She also made small but significant lifestyle changes such as parking at the far end of the supermarket parking lot. After several months of this, she noticed that her lunchtime walk had become an important way of helping her "de-stress" before the afternoon at work, and that if she did not get out for a walk at all she started to feel like a "caged tiger." By sticking diligently to her planned walking goals over an extended period of time, this patient had managed to incorporate them into her normal daily routine to such an extent that not being active became an unattractive option.

A patient whose work involved looking after a booth at trade fairs, made a habit of walking around the booth regularly rather than sitting passively beside it. Another patient found that putting on some music and having a dance in her living room was not only good exercise but also served as a mood lifter.

Step 6: Maintaining the Increase in Activity

As with the changes in eating, a major goal is that the changes in activity are maintained in the long term. Thus, once addressed, activity needs to remain a focus of treatment right up to the end. Potential (or actual) barriers to the maintenance of the increase in activity need to be addressed, as does the need to restart being active following times when the new pattern has been disrupted (for example, after illness, during the winter, or following vacations).

Increasing Formal Exercise

Many people with obesity find formal exercise difficult and aversive. This is understandable, as their weight and size may impair their performance. Other reasons for their dislike of exercise include body image concerns and difficulty finding appropriate clothing.

Although increasing the amount of formal exercise is not a goal of this treatment, it should be encouraged if the patient is sympathetic to the idea. Although not needed for weight loss, it will improve the patient's physical health.

The topic of formal exercise will have been raised in the assessment of activity levels. The therapist should ask patients about their attitude to various forms of formal exercise (see step 4 above). If the patient is interested in exercising, the pros and cons of these forms of exercise should be discussed, together with possible obstacles to the patient's participation in them. These might include lack of availability of the necessary resources (e.g., a swimming pool or gym), the need for special clothing or equipment (e.g., running shoes or a tracksuit), and sensitivity about being seen exercising. All such obstacles should be addressed sensitively using a problem-solving approach (see Chapter 4). Means of facilitating exercise should be discussed, but not in a way that puts pressure on the patient. Suggestions might include exercising with a family member or friend, joining a health club or gym, and buying equipment for exercising at home (e.g., a stationary bicycle or a rowing machine).

As with lifestyle activity, specific incremental targets may be set and reviewed at subsequent sessions. It is especially important to praise patients for any efforts to exercise, however modest they might seem. With patients who are unwilling to exercise at their present weight, the topic may be put aside and revisited later on in treatment.

The United States National Institutes of Health has published information for overweight people interested in integrating physical activity into their lives. It is titled "Active at Any Size" and is available on-line at http://www.niddk.nih.gov under the heading "Weight Loss and Control."

CHAPTER 7

Module V: Addressing Body Image Concerns

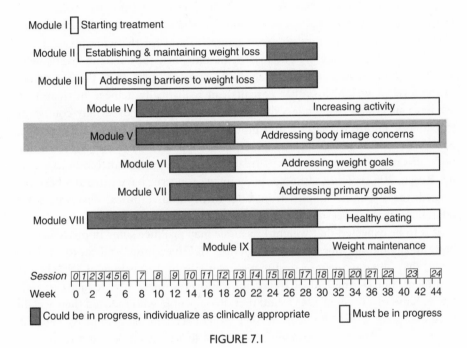

FIGURE 7.1

Body image refers to an individual's perception of his or her body as well as attitude toward appearance. It is subjective rather than objective. An individual's perception may not accord with the views of others, indeed it is very often more negative than the judgments of others. Body image concerns can constitute a major obstacle to weight maintenance. The goals of this module are as follows:

1. To provide education about the role of body image in weight control and the development and maintenance of body image concerns.
2. To identify body image concerns.
3. To address these concerns.
4. To encourage the development of a positive body image.

The Role of Body Image in Weight Loss

Concerns about appearance are extremely common, particularly among women in Western societies. Indeed, they have been referred to as "normative discontent" (Rodin, Silberstein & Striegel-Moore, 1984). In such Western societies, being overweight is generally viewed as physically unattractive. Consequently, many overweight people dislike their appearance, and this is often the main reason they seek to lose weight. They believe that weight loss will improve their appearance and attractiveness, and that as a result they will feel better about themselves (see Rosen, 2002). The perception that being overweight is unattractive appears to account for the low goal weights that many obese people set for themselves (see Chapter 8) and for the widespread dissatisfaction with moderate weight loss if, despite this, they remain overweight. Thus body image concerns are likely to be a major obstacle to the acceptance of the level of weight loss that patients can realistically achieve in treatment. We have suggested that undervaluing the weight loss achieved may contribute to patients' failure to acquire and practice weight maintenance skills (Cooper & Fairburn, 2001, 2002). This suggestion is supported by the observation that body dissatisfaction at the end of treatment appears to predict weight regain (cf. Rosen, 2002). Thus, although body image concerns have generally been neglected, there is some support from both theory and empirical observation for addressing these concerns during treatment for obesity.

It is to be expected that weight loss alone may produce some improvement in body image among obese people. Collins, McCabe, Jupp, and Sutton (1983) found that obese women overestimated their size by an average of 19% before treatment, but by the end of treatment the overestimate was reduced to only 8.8%. Similarly, Cash (1994) found that obese people who reduced their weight by 24% using a very-low-calorie diet experienced marked improvements in most aspects of body image. However, weight loss by itself does not remove all body image problems, particularly if the weight loss is only moderate. For example, Cash, Counts, and Huffine (1990) compared three groups of people: average-weight people who had never been overweight, average-weight people who had been overweight, and people who were currently overweight. The formerly overweight subjects were found to be similar in their attitude to their appearance to the currently overweight group. Compared to those who had never been overweight, they were less satisfied with their bodies, and they perceived themselves as fatter. Moreover, weight reduction may not be necessary to bring about improvements in body image. For example, some obese people are able to combat their distressing preoccupation with appearance through cognitive-behavioral "body image therapy," without losing weight at all (Rosen, Orosan, & Reiter, 1995).

We suggest that work on body image has an important place in the overall management of obese people. Although some patients with obesity have little or no concern about appearance, and so do not need help in this area, others have major body image problems that are complex, deep-seated, and a major source of distress. Ideally such work should be tailored to the individual, rather than presented in a group format, as people's needs vary greatly.

In this cognitive-behavioral treatment, therapeutic work on body image occurs in parallel with a focus on weight goals (including "acceptance," see Chapter 8) and primary goals (see Chapter 9). It is important to address these areas simultaneously, and over a substantial period of time (in our practice, the focus on body image is introduced at any point from week 8 onward and may be revisited as often as necessary until the end of treatment), in order to achieve changes in these patients' goals and self-image in enough time for these to be tested, modified, and consolidated. Body image issues continue to be addressed during the period of weight maintenance, when the patient is no longer trying to lose any weight (see Chapter 11), with the aim of tackling any residual body image problems which might remain at the new weight.

Determining When to Enter the Body Image Module

Weight loss should be well established before this module is entered; indeed, it may be beginning to slow down. We have used the following guidelines (see Figure 7.1):

1. It may be entered from week 8 onward in those patients with prominent body image concerns (especially if unhappiness with their body shape leads to overeating).
2. It should be entered by the middle of treatment at the latest. (Our practice has been to always enter this module by week 20.)

Therapists should explain that they would like to start to discuss the patient's feelings and attitudes toward their appearance adding, if necessary, that these are often relevant to successful weight maintenance in the long term.

Overview of Module V

The module consists of a brief introduction to the topic, followed by several partially independent sections. The first concerns assessment, and it involves the completion of a body image checklist. The second is educational and is relevant to all patients. The remaining sections describe a range of procedures, each of which involves examining thoughts, beliefs, and behaviors in an objective way. Such objective examination allows patients to separate and distance themselves from their thoughts and decrease the behavior that contributes to them. The choice of procedures to use and the order in which to implement them should depend on the needs of individual patients. For some patients (particularly those with severe or longstanding problems) therapeutic work on these issues will need to continue over a number of weeks. Each section includes suggested interventions with related homework assignments. These assignments require following up in subsequent sessions. As noted earlier, the focus on body image should run in parallel with other aspects of treatment (for example, the work on weight goals and the addressing of other primary goals; see Chapters 8 and 9 respectively).

Introduction: The Concept of Body Image as Distinct from Physical Appearance

Therapists should explain to patients that what is meant by body image is not a person's actual (objective) physical appearance but his or her view or "mental picture" of his or her body. In other words, it is how they think and feel about their body. Possible examples to illustrate the difference between a person's body image and actual physical appearance may include the following (choose examples that are of relevance to the particular patient):

- Feeling fat or overweight during early teenage years, even if not objectively overweight
- A person who looks good (or at least unremarkable) but who is concerned about some physical feature, such as baldness, facial appearance, or figure
- In contrast, someone who is overweight yet who is confident and feels good about his or her body

Therapists should also explain that many people are dissatisfied with at least some aspect of their appearance and might like to change the way they look. However, this dissatisfaction does not usually interfere with their overall view of themselves as being adequate or worthwhile, nor does it affect their ability to socialize or work. For other people, however, body image concerns do affect their overall view of themselves and their everyday functioning. The therapist should go on to discuss with patients the extent to which this does or does not apply to them.

Assessment: Identifying Body Image Concerns

The first step in addressing body image involves an assessment of the extent and nature of the patient's concerns. To this end patients should complete a body image checklist (see Table 7.1; Handout M). The therapist should explain that some of the questions on the checklist are quite personal, but the patient should answer them as frankly as possible. The checklist can be completed either as homework (if the therapist thinks that this will not cause the patient too much distress) or, particularly in cases where patients are very distressed by their appearance, with the therapist during the session.

After the checklist has been completed, the therapist should review it in detail with the patient in order to agree on particular problem areas. In our experience

TABLE 7.1

The Body Image Checklist

Instructions: Please answer these questions as they have applied to you over the PAST 4 WEEKS. Please place a tick in the appropriate column.

Over the past 4 weeks ...	Not at all	Sometimes	Frequently	Not applicable
Questions about avoidance:				
Have you avoided seeing yourself in mirrors (or window reflections)?				
Have you avoided weighing yourself?				
Have you dressed in a way to disguise your appearance?				
Have you avoided your shape being seen by others (e.g., swimming pools, communal changing rooms, etc.)?				
Have you avoided taking part in physical activities because of your shape?				
Have you avoided shopping for clothes?				
Have you avoided being seen at home naked (e.g., when undressing or bathing)?				
Have you avoided wearing clothes that show the shape of your body?				
Have you avoided (or limited) close physical contact because of your dislike of your shape (e.g., shaking hands, sexual contact, hugging, kissing)?				
Have you avoided wearing clothes that show your skin (e.g., short-sleeve shirts, shorts)?				
Have you avoided social occasions because of your shape?				
Questions about checking:				
Have you studied your overall appearance in the mirror?				
Have you studied parts of your body in the mirror?				
Have you weighed yourself?				
Have you measured parts of your body?				
Have you assessed your size in other ways?				
Have you pinched yourself to see how much fat there is?				
General questions:				
Have you felt unhappy about your shape?				
Have you worried about the size of particular parts of your body?				
Have you worried about your body wobbling?				
Have you felt ashamed or embarrassed about your body in public?				
Have you felt that other people were noticing your shape?				
Have you felt that your body was disgusting?				
Have you thought that other people were being critical of you because of your shape?				
Have you felt that you take up too much room (e.g., when sitting on a sofa or bus seat)?				
Have you sought reassurance that your shape is not as bad as you think it is?				
Have people made critical comments about your shape or appearance?				

many patients with obesity are highly sensitive about such issues, and this will often be the first time that they have talked about them. It is therefore important that this review is done in a sympathetic and accepting manner. It should not be rushed.

This review will result in the therapist's having a better understanding of the patient's body image concerns. It will also help to identify which area it is most important to target first. The overall aim is to help patients learn to accept their appearance and themselves. This is important because people who are unable to accept their new weight and appearance seem to have difficulty both implementing and adhering to weight maintenance strategies with the result that they are prone to regain the lost weight. This point should be explained to the patient. The therapist should also stress that addressing body image issues will be done in conjunction with continuing work on weight loss (because it is important not to give patients the impression that attempts to improve their body image are to be a substitute for weight loss). If it is apparent that the patient does not have significant body image concerns, there is no need to proceed further with this module.

When reviewing the body image checklist, a patient mentioned that she was reluctant to go swimming. This was an activity she had enjoyed when she was younger, and she wished to resume. There were good grounds for pursuing this matter in treatment, as it was relevant to her body image, primary goals, and activity levels. The therapist and patient discussed her concerns and set relevant step-by-step homework, such that the patient did go swimming and began to feel reasonably comfortable about it. However, the patient reported that she still felt very uncomfortable about changing in a communal area and always sought a private cubicle. The therapist questioned her about this, to see if it was an issue that warranted further attention. The patient explained that she felt self-conscious because she had been brought up to believe that it was not "proper" to get undressed in front of other people, rather than due to any specific concerns about her body shape or size. She explained that once she was in her bathing suit she did not feel embarrassed and was happy to continue swimming. The therapist did not therefore pursue this, as it appeared to be an issue of cultural "norms" rather than a specific body image concern, and it did not result in functional impairment.

Personalized Education about Body Image

In this educational section, three topics are addressed: the development of a negative body image, the maintenance of a negative body image, and ways of modifying a negative body image.

The Development of a Negative Body Image

With those patients who have significant body image concerns, the therapist should devote some time to discussing the development and, more importantly, the maintenance of body image problems. This discussion should include consideration of how the various etiological processes might have operated in their particular case.

To start with, the therapist should explain that four processes contribute to the development of a negative body image.

1. *General social pressures.* These are social pressures to conform to a particular standard for physical attractiveness. For example, in the West today, thinness and a well-toned body are valued for women, whereas tallness and muscularity are valued for men. Being overweight is viewed negatively for both men and women. Other societies have different standards for attractiveness (for example, being overweight is valued as a sign of prosperity and health in some countries). Over the years fashions have evolved even in our own society (e.g., the large women depicted in 15th- to 18th-century art, and the curvaceous film stars of the 1940s and 1950s), indicating that there is nothing intrinsically attractive about our current norms. The problem is that cultural norms for physical attractiveness are restrictive and difficult (or even impossible) for many people to attain. Women are under particular pressure to conform to the currently favored appearance and are rewarded socially for doing so (e.g., by a process of "positive stereotyping," they may be viewed as more intelligent, more competent, and more in control). As a result, their self-image is often strongly associated with the way they view their appearance.

2. *Patient-specific social pressures.* These are social pressures particular to the individual patient that have magnified the general social pressure to be slim. For example, the patient may have been brought up in a family in which there was particular interest in appearance, or they may have other family members who are slim and with whom they have been unfavorably compared. They may have worked in environments in which there were intense pressures not to be overweight (e.g., in certain sales jobs).

3. *Physical distinctiveness.* Some people attract more attention than others because their appearance is distinctive in some way. For example, an early or late puberty may have resulted in a patient standing out as being different from her or his peers. Being especially tall or short, or having acne or any other distinctive physical feature, may also result in unwanted attention or teasing from others.

4. *Critical incidents in the past.* These are specific negative incidents that have contributed to the formation of the patient's negative body image; for example, being teased at school for being overweight, being humiliated by a sports teacher, or being told by a partner or doctor that one is "fat."

This discussion should be relatively brief but personalized to the particular patient. Thus patients should be asked whether such processes and events have applied to them. The aim is to develop an understanding of how their body image concerns have arisen. It is important that not too much time is devoted to the development of the patient's body image concerns, because it is their maintenance that is of greater importance to treatment.

The Maintenance of a Negative Body Image

The discussion of the development of body image problems forms a useful introduction to the topic of their maintenance. Therapists should explain that some degree of understanding of how the patient's body image concerns arose is interesting and valuable, but the crucial issue is what keeps them going. It is these maintaining processes that need to be addressed in order to overcome the body image problem.

The therapist should describe the following maintaining processes. The emphasis in the discussion should be on establishing whether they are relevant to the patient and, if so, how much influence they have. (The review of the patient's body image checklist will already have highlighted many of these factors.)

1. Maintaining Factors in the Environment

General Social Pressures.   It should be pointed out to patients that, were they living in a society in which being large was considered attractive, it is unlikely that they would have body image concerns. Living in a society that values thinness serves to perpetuate a negative body image.

Patient-Specific Social Pressures.   The patient may be exposed to particular pressures not to be her or his present shape. The patient's job may raise specific difficulties (e.g., public presentations; traveling on buses or airplanes) or the family environment may pose particular problems (e.g., a partner or child may make negative comments about her or his appearance). Such ongoing social pressures may contribute to the maintenance of the patient's negative body image.

2. Maintaining Behavior

Body Avoidance.   This refers to the avoidance of situations in which patients fear they will feel particularly self-conscious about their appearance. Examples include shopping for clothes, participating in certain sports (e.g., swimming or tennis) or other physical activities (e.g., dancing), having sexual relationships, and attending social occasions. It also includes avoiding weighing themselves. Therapists should explain that, while avoiding situations may avoid distress and discomfort in the short term (e.g., distress at seeing one's body while trying on clothes; distress that one cannot fit into certain clothes; discomfort at being seen in certain situations), it does not allow patients to feel less anxious or negative about the situation. Rather, it perpetuates it. Avoidance prevents patients from learning that the feared consequences (such as being exposed to public ridicule, or discovering that they cannot fit into certain clothes) often do not materialize. In some cases avoidance may also magnify the body image concerns by reinforcing the patient's belief that his or her body is so unacceptable that it is necessary to go to great lengths to hide it. It also does not let patients learn to deal with the feared consequences should they occur.

Body Checking. Among some people with obesity, the opposite occurs and they engage in repeated body checking. This involves frequent checking of aspects of appearance or weight (e.g., studying oneself in mirrors and scrutinizing parts of the body, measuring body dimensions, pinching skin folds, repeatedly asking for reassurance about appearance, frequent weighing). The therapist should explain how body checking of this type tends to maintain body image concerns because it keeps the target of dissatisfaction under scrutiny. Although there may be short-term relief gained from such checking, it does not last. Rather, body checking maintains a negative body image by increasing preoccupation with the focus of the concern and by perpetuating the idea that constant checking is needed in order to prevent the feared consequence (e.g., increased "fatness" or weight gain).

3. Maintaining Thoughts and Beliefs

Negative Predictions. Patients with body image concerns tend to make negative predictions about their appearance, which serve to maintain these concerns. Examples include predictions such as:

- I must disguise my hips; everyone will see how fat they are.
- People will think I look ridiculous in sports clothes.
- There is no point buying nice clothes or having my hair done because I will still look fat and that is what people will notice.
- No one would want to employ me looking the way I do.
- People do not take me seriously because I am overweight.

The therapist should explain that body image concerns lead to systematic biases in perception and thinking (e.g., selectively looking in the mirror at body parts that are viewed as particularly "fat" rather than also looking at the whole body in context; overestimating the likelihood of negative reactions from others; or focusing only on weight and shape, while discounting other positive qualities). Such biases make it likely that patients will accept their negative predictions as true and act accordingly. As a result these biases are likely to encourage a variety of forms of body avoidance and checking, which prevent the patient from finding out whether the feared consequences that they predict actually occur.

Recurrent Critical Thoughts.   Critical thoughts about appearance or weight are a part of body image concerns and serve to maintain them. Examples include thoughts such as:

- I look so awful.
- I am fat and unattractive.
- My hips and bottom are too big.
- I never look good.
- I look like a massive blob.

The therapist should explain that recurrent critical thoughts about appearance such as these play an important role in maintaining a negative body image because they (like negative predictions) tend to be accepted as true. As they are self-critical, they are distressing and often lead to further negative or biased interpretations of information about body shape or weight, or to unhelpful behavior (e.g., failing to notice the positive effects of weight loss and concluding instead that nothing will make any difference as one will always be fat and unattractive; or comfort eating as a way of coping with such thoughts).

4. Misinterpreting Physical Stimuli

Certain physical stimuli may be interpreted as evidence of fatness or weight gain. One example is the sensation of body wobble. Most women's bodies wobble to some degree. This is a normal female characteristic, yet some obese women interpret it as being indicative of fatness. This is a powerful maintaining factor because it operates each time the person is aware of wobbling (potentially every time a step is taken). Similarly, but less powerfully, premenstrual fluid retention may be misinterpreted as evidence of increasing fatness. Such issues should be discussed if they appear to be of particular relevance to the patient.

5. Dysfunctional Beliefs

Often negative predictions and recurrent critical thoughts about appearance are a reflection of a more general dysfunctional belief or attitude that is maintaining body image concerns. Examples include beliefs such as:

- Success depends on being thin.
- Only thin people have successful relationships.
- I will only have self-confidence if I am thin.
- To be attractive, I have to be thin.
- No one will respect me unless I am thin.
- To be popular, I need to be thin.
- I cannot get on with my life until I am thin.

Such attitudes may emerge when patients talk about why they would like to lose weight, or how they think life would be different if they achieved their goal weight. Again these attitudes tend to be accepted without questioning and as such serve to maintain body image dissatisfaction because they encourage the belief that it is the patient's appearance that is primarily responsible for difficulties such as poor self-confidence and relationship problems. Additionally they may encourage patients to delay attempts to improve their relationships or improve their self-confidence until they have lost weight. For a further discussion of this, see Chapter 9.

Having identified which (if any) of these maintaining processes are operating, therapists should summarize the discussion and explain that future sessions will be devoted to planning and practicing change in these areas.

Monitoring Body Image Concerns

The starting point in addressing body image concerns is monitoring them. To this end, the patient should be asked to start completing a body image record (Handout N). They should record instances when:

- they are aware that they were thinking critically about their body;
- they avoid situations because of the way they feel about their body;
- they check their body in an inappropriate way.

They should record the details of each situation, their emotions, thoughts, and beliefs (if relevant) and behavior, as well as any consequences. To help them do this, the therapist should review some example records (Table 7.2, 7.3, and 7.4; Handouts O, P, and Q), which should be given to the patient as guidelines about how to record.

The patient should be encouraged to record two or three examples before the next appointment. The final column ("alternative thoughts") can be left blank the first week that the patient completes these records (unless he or she is able to come up with alternatives), but in subsequent sessions, the patient should be encouraged to attempt to complete this column as well.

Some patients return having not completed any body image records. The reasons for this need to be explored. They include the following:

- Uncertainty over what was required. The therapist should clarify exactly what the patient is expected to do and the reasons for doing it.
- Embarrassment about such thoughts or behaviors. This possibility should be raised and the therapist should try dispel the patient's concerns.
- The absence of relevant thoughts or behaviors. This is possible but it should be sensitively challenged especially if such features had been reported on the body image checklist. If there were no examples of problematic thoughts or behaviors in the past week, the patient should be encouraged to record any that occur before the following session. If there really do appear to be no body image difficulties, there is no need to continue with this module, although it is useful to return to the topic occasionally to ensure that it continues not to be a problem.
- Resistance to the task. This can be difficult to overcome. The rationale for addressing body image should be restated.

TABLE 7.2

A Completed Body Image Diary—Example 1: Avoidance

Record on the body image diary times when: you were thinking negatively about your body; you avoided situations because of the way you felt about your body; you were checking your body in an inappropriate way.

Situation	Feelings	Thoughts	Behavior	Consequences	Alternative thoughts
Being asked by my child to accompany him on a bike ride.	Anxious about what to say, sad and miserable about the situation.	The whole street will see me looking ridiculous on a bicycle. I will wobble. I cannot ride my bike until my body looks better. This is another thing I cannot do because of the way I look.	Told my son that I could not go. Made up an excuse (lied).	Not able to do things with my son, always putting things off until I get thinner.	It is me who thinks I will look ridiculous and disgusting. I am assuming everyone will think this; I do not actually know what everyone thinks. In the past I have been surprised that people have not always been thinking what I thought they were—in this case perhaps I could find out. If I saw someone who was overweight riding a bicycle I would not think they looked ridiculous—I would think it was healthy exercise. So why do I have to wait until I lose weight? Other people seem to be able to do it who are even heavier than me. Besides, I used to enjoy riding a bicycle, and it is good exercise. By saying I cannot do it, I will deprive myself of the opportunity of doing exercise that might make me feel better about myself. I should try to ride and find out what happens.

108

TABLE 7.3

A Completed Body Image Diary—Example 2: Repeated Checking

Record on the body image diary times when: you were thinking negatively about your body; you were feeling negatively about your body; you avoided situations because of the way you felt about your body; you were checking your body in an inappropriate way.

Situation	Feelings	Thoughts	Behavior	Consequences	Alternative thoughts
Getting dressed in the morning.	Really miserable, disgusted and angry with myself.	My hips and bottom are so big. I do not look nice in these clothes—in fact nothing looks good on me. I always look terrible.	I try on several outfits in the hope that they will hide my hips and bottom. I check myself in the mirror several times and from all angles to see if I look any better. I eventually choose an outfit that is slightly better, but not much.	Once again, I'm late for work because it takes so long to dress, and I still spend all day worrying about how I look. I repeatedly go to the restroom to check myself in the mirror—still don't like what I see. When I buy clothes, I only consider whether they will hide my hips and bottom—I don't bother considering anything else.	Rationally, I know my shape cannot really have changed noticeably overnight. I felt OK at work yesterday, so the fact that I feel low today is not because I am fatter, but because I am upset about something else. My colleagues are not going to be watching me to see if my shape has changed overnight, but they will notice if I'm late for work. I know that anyone who scrutinizes themselves in a mirror could find things about their appearance that they want to change. Constantly examining myself in the mirror just makes me feel worse especially as I only look at the bits I hate—I don't bother about my hair and eyes, which are OK. So I will try to stop doing that. I am doing what I can to help myself—I have already lost some weight, although it has been slower than I would like. Now I will just make the best of where I am at the moment. I may try buying some new clothes that I feel really good in.

TABLE 7.4

A Completed Body Image Diary—Example 3: Negative Thoughts

Record on the body image diary times when: you were thinking negatively about your body; you avoided situations because of the way you felt about your body; you were checking your body in an inappropriate way.

Situation	Feelings	Thoughts	Behavior	Consequences	Alternative thoughts
Sitting in dentist's waiting room looking at clothes in a fashion magazine.	Envious of models looking good in great clothes, miserable and disgusted with my body.	I never look good in clothes. I cannot fit into any decent clothes any way. It is not fair; the women in the magazine are so thin and attractive, and my body is so fat and ugly.	Felt so bad I bought a bar of chocolate on the way home to console myself.	Felt even worse later because eating chocolate will make me even fatter and make the situation worse.	Just because I am not thin and perfect like a model does not mean that I am unattractive. I know people whom I regard as attractive and they don't look like models. I am comparing myself to an ideal no one can attain—photographs of models are touched up to remove imperfections.
					I always compare myself to people whom I think are more attractive than I am, and not to those who are less attractive. If someone else did that, I would think they were being unfair. Perhaps I am being unduly hard on myself because I never think of the things I am good at. I know that society's ideals for shape are narrow, and I admire people who are not so influenced by them. Thinking the way I do is not helpful, because it results in my eating the wrong things, which only makes things worse.
					Although I weigh more than I would like to, this does not mean that I am totally unattractive or that I cannot look stylish.

Once the patient has completed some body image records, the therapist should review one or two in detail to begin to illustrate how the patient's behavior and thoughts may be maintaining his or her negative body image. At this stage it is best to concentrate principally on the behaviors that appear to be maintaining the problem, although thoughts and beliefs should be noted for later discussion. Then, depending on the nature of the problems identified, body avoidance, body checking, and maintaining thoughts should each be addressed as relevant (see below).

Addressing Avoidance of Body Shape

Rationale for Tackling Body Shape Avoidance

Avoiding situations that cause distress (or are predicted to cause distress) tends to perpetuate negative feelings and thoughts. Although avoiding such situations may prevent distress and discomfort in the short term, it does not allow patients to gain reliable information about their body shape, nor to learn to feel less anxious or negative about their situation. Rather it results in patients' being dependent on subjective (almost always negative) judgments about how they or others will feel, and as a consequence they are not able to disconfirm their worst fears.

The therapist should illustrate these processes by reviewing examples from the patients' own experience (obtained either from their body image record as described above or from the body image checklist). The aim is to illustrate how avoidance is contributing to their body image concerns.

This preparatory discussion should culminate in the conclusion that the best way of addressing avoidance (and its consequences) is to expose oneself to the distressing situations, test out one's predictions, and address any adverse consequences.

Procedure

Once the patient has understood and accepted the rationale for tackling avoidance, the patient and therapist should make detailed plans for addressing it. The key steps are as follows:

1. The patient and therapist should agree on a specific and well-defined behavioral task (e.g., to eliminate a form of avoidance altogether or to phase it out gradually over some weeks).
2. The task should be one the patient is likely to achieve.
3. The patient should be encouraged to anticipate or predict the likely consequences (both behavioral and cognitive) of engaging in the task.
4. The patient and therapist should plan the steps required to achieve the task and plan how to cope with anticipated difficulties.

5. The patient should record attempts to perform the task on his or her monitoring records together with associated thoughts both before and after.

6. At the next session the outcome should be reviewed with the emphasis being on whether the actual outcome was as predicted by the patient. Positive aspects of the outcome should be emphasized (including the fact of having actually tried it), as well as what the patient has learned as a result.

Although she had achieved reasonable weight loss, a patient described avoiding buying clothes and having her hair styled because she was so dissatisfied with her appearance. In discussion she was able to see that although she was thereby succeeding in avoiding negative feelings about her body, it also maintained her belief that she looked bad. In addition, it resulted in her wearing clothes she did not like and her hair being "in a mess," which also supported her view of herself as fat and unattractive. On successfully addressing this avoidance, she discovered that she did not feel worse about her body, as she had predicted, but instead she felt better. She also received compliments about how stylish she looked.

When discussing body image, it became apparent that a patient had many forms of avoidance. The therapist asked her to list these, then rank them to help them decide where to start. The patient suggested that the one she would be most willing to tackle initially would be her avoidance of seeing herself in mirrors. The therapist restated the rationale for tackling avoidance, and suggested that the patient pick a time when she could look at herself in front of a full-length mirror. The plan was that, in advance of doing so, she spend time writing down what she expected to think and feel, and what she believed would happen as a consequence of looking in the mirror. The therapist also asked her to write down afterward what she had actually thought and felt, and what the consequences of the exercise were.

The patient completed this exercise and reported back on it. She stated that she had predicted that she would look in the mirror and see a "massive blob" and that this would feel totally abhorrent to her. In fact she had found that although the physical image did not delight her, it was not totally abhorrent. However, it was the ensuing train of thoughts that had upset her badly. She saw her physical imperfection as being indicative of weakness in other areas of her life.

Given the focus of the treatment, the therapist decided to focus on the body image aspect of this experience and to highlight the positive aspect of what had happened—namely that the patient's physical image was not nearly as bad as she had predicted.

The therapist said, "I notice that what you predicted was different from what actually happened when you looked in the mirror. That is important to remember. Maybe there are other instances where what you predict would not necessarily be the case. If we could identify these we might be able to help you feel more positive about your weight and shape."

Where avoidance is a problem, the issue should be repeatedly addressed until the patient is able to comfortably do the things that were previously avoided. Body image records need to be completed each week to indicate how the patient is progressing in this respect.

Addressing Body Checking

Rationale for Tackling Body Checking

The therapist should discuss with patients how body checking focuses attention on sources of dissatisfaction and usually increases preoccupation with them. An analogy can be drawn with a teenager looking at a blemish on her face, and finding that the more attention is directed at the blemish, the larger and more prominent it seems. While body checking may in some instances provide reassurance, this generally does not last. Rather it provides unreliable information that is often influenced by extraneous variables such as mood states and the patient's expectations. This information, which is usually interpreted negatively, tends to maintain and sometimes even increase the patient's body dissatisfaction. It also reinforces the belief that body checking is needed to prevent feared consequences from occurring.

The therapist should illustrate these processes by reviewing examples from the patient's experience (obtained either from his or her body image record or from the body image checklist). The aim is to illustrate how body checking is contributing to body image concerns.

This preparatory discussion should culminate in the conclusion that the best way of addressing dysfunctional body checking (and its consequences) is to stop doing it, test out the patient's predictions, and address any adverse consequences. In parallel with reducing dysfunctional checking, the patient should be encouraged to develop "normal" body checking habits. This involves agreeing what is normal in this regard. In general this involves a discussion about the appropriate use of mirrors, covering topics such as the purpose of looking in the mirror, the frequency of doing so and the time spent looking. Patients should be encouraged to look in mirrors to establish that they look alright generally and that their clothes are in place and when doing so they should look briefly at their whole body in perspective, rather than spend a long time scrutinizing specific disliked body parts.

Procedure

Once the patient has understood and accepted the rationale for addressing the body checking, the patient and therapist should make detailed plans for tackling it. The key steps are the same in principle as those used to tackle avoidance:

1. The patient and therapist should agree on a specific and well-defined behavioral task (e.g., to eliminate a form of body checking altogether or to phase it out gradually over some weeks). If appropriate it should be agreed that the checking should be replaced with "normal checking."
2. The task should be one which the patient is likely to achieve.
3. The patient should be encouraged to anticipate the likely consequences (both behavioral and cognitive) of engaging in the task.
4. The patient and therapist should plan the steps required to achieve the task and plan how to cope with anticipated difficulties. If appropriate, a plan should be made for "normal" checking.
5. The patient should record on the monitoring records attempts to perform the task together with associated thoughts both before and after.
6. At the next session the patient and therapist should review the outcome with the emphasis being on whether the actual outcome was as predicted by the patient. Positive aspects of the outcome should be emphasized (including the fact of having actually tried it) as well as what the patient has learned as a result.

A patient who was finding it difficult to lose further weight, having already lost 10% of her original weight, was reluctant to consider maintaining her new weight because she felt her hips were still unacceptably large. She described taking an extremely long time to dress each morning because she had to try on several skirts and dresses and check her appearance in the mirror to find out which one best disguised her hips. While doing this she also assessed whether her hips had increased in size, by assessing the tightness of her clothes.

After discussion, the patient agreed that it was possible that repeatedly checking her hips and attempting to disguise them was increasing her negative views on her body. She agreed, somewhat reluctantly, to find out what would happen if she resisted the body checking on one occasion. The patient thought she would be able to achieve this by not allowing sufficient time before work to complete her checking and clothes changing. Instead, she would dress, check her appearance briefly in the mirror taking care to look at her whole body (not just her hips), and leave for work. She predicted that this would result in her being even more preoccupied than usual with how she looked and that, if she continued not to check over the next few weeks, her hips were bound to get bigger.

When the patient and therapist reviewed the outcome of this experiment, the patient reported that although she had been worried about her hips as she was traveling to work, her overall level of preoccupation during the day was no worse than usual. This persuaded her to continue the experiment. After a few weeks, she reported that her overall level of preoccupation with thoughts about her hips had declined and her hips were no larger.

Another patient described pinching the fat around her stomach (particularly when standing in front of mirrors), and checking the fat at the back of her neck. The therapist elicited a detailed description of the behavior, and asked the patient to describe what she was thinking and how she felt when she checked her body in this way. The patient found that it tended to induce negative feelings, particularly when she used it to confirm her belief that she was "fatter" that day. The therapist discussed the notion that such checking is unhelpful because it tends to reinforce negative beliefs about the body through focusing on the source of dissatisfaction and perpetuating the idea that checking is necessary in order to prevent weight gain. The patient agreed that body pinching is not an objective measure of fatness and is generally unhelpful.

Having reviewed the issue and observed how checking was unhelpful, the patient decided to stop. She found that stopping the checking of her stomach was straightforward, and she simply stopped from that point on. However she found it more difficult to stop checking her neck. She needed to remind herself each time she found herself checking that it was not helpful and that she only continued to do it out of habit. When she caught herself touching her neck to check it, she snapped her fingers instead, forming a new incompatible habit. Over a period of weeks, she was able to completely stop checking the fat on her neck, and she then stopped snapping her fingers as well.

Addressing Social Pressures

Living in a society that values thinness tends to perpetuate the negative body image of many of those with obesity. In addition there may be certain patient-specific social pressures, which will already have been identified (e.g., family attitudes or job requirements). There is little the patient can do to alter the general social pressure to be thin, and it may also be difficult to modify the patient-specific social pressures. Nevertheless it is helpful for patients to be aware of these pressures and their unfairness for people who are not naturally thin. Therapists should encourage patients to question whether criticism and negative reactions from others are justified or are simply a result of society's negative stereotypes about obesity. In other words, patients should ask themselves, "Is this a problem with me, or is this a problem with them (or with this society) because they hold a prejudice?" If the problem is judged to be with the other person or with a judgmental society, patients may not be able to do anything to change the prejudiced view, but they may decide not to let such prejudice leave them feeling bad about themselves. The goal is to help them distance themselves from pressures to conform to such stereotypes. Patients and therapists should also work together to find ways of coping with such prejudice (e.g., ignoring it, writing an angry letter to a local newspaper, joining a society that campaigns against prejudice, etc.).

Addressing Maintaining Thoughts and Beliefs

Rationale for Tackling Problematic Thoughts and Beliefs

Therapists should remind patients about the role of thoughts and beliefs in maintaining body image concerns, using examples from the patient's body image diary. These include negative predictions, recurrent critical thoughts, misinterpretation of bodily stimuli, and dysfunctional beliefs. The attribution of weight-independent difficulties to the weight problem is a related issue, which will be discussed in more detail in Chapter 9. If applicable, therapists should remind patients that some of the thoughts that have led to their body avoidance or checking have already been identified and challenged indirectly by behaving differently and observing the consequences.

Procedures for Addressing Problematic Thoughts and Beliefs

Therapists should explain that it is helpful to examine thoughts and beliefs in an objective way. Such examination enables patients to separate and distance themselves from their thoughts and assess whether they are accurate or helpful. The first step in doing this is to learn to identify these thoughts and the contexts in which they occur. The thoughts and beliefs can be identified from four main sources:

- Negative thoughts recorded in the body image diary
- Negative thoughts already identified that led to body avoidance or checking
- Concerns the patient has expressed about accepting a higher weight than her or his original weight goal
- Concerns expressed by the patient when failing to lose weight or when weight loss has slowed or ceased

It is particularly helpful to identify and work with commonly recurring thoughts (rather than isolated thoughts) because they are likely to express those problematic or self-defeating beliefs that particularly require modification.

Having identified one or more problematic thoughts, the therapist should introduce ways of questioning and reevaluating these thoughts and beliefs using standard cognitive techniques. Therapists who are unfamiliar with these techniques may find it helpful to read the account by Beck (1995). A useful source of reference for therapists in the area of body image problems is Cash (1996). There is also a self-help book for patients (Cash, 1997).

Briefly, there are a number of ways in which patients can be helped to re-examine their thoughts and beliefs. These include the following:

Reviewing Evidence and Finding Alternative Perspectives

Patients should be encouraged to examine the evidence for their negative predictions and self-critical thoughts. The therapist should help them to consider evidence that supports their predictions and thoughts, as well as evidence that does not. Patients should also be encouraged to actively seek alternative perspectives from the one they hold. The aim is to help patients arrive at a more balanced conclusion about the accuracy of their negative predictions and self-critical thoughts.

A patient, who in the course of body image work had begun wearing shorter skirts, reported a telephone conversation with her mother that she had found distressing. Her mother had said that if the patient were going to wear a short skirt, she should wear thick tights. This immediately made the patient feel more self-conscious about wearing a short skirt and resulted in her wanting to cover her legs. She concluded that her mother thought her legs were fat and horrible and that her mother was right in thinking that other people would not wish to see them.

The therapist encouraged the patient to examine the evidence for her interpretation of the situation and also encouraged her to consider alternative perspectives. The patient was able to question her interpretation of her mother's comments by noting that her mother had not seen her for several months (during which time the patient had lost weight) and therefore could not know what she looked like in a short skirt. She realized that she did not know what her mother had meant by this remark and decided to find out by asking. When asked, it appeared that her mother thought she should cover her legs because they were not tanned rather than because there was anything wrong with their shape. The patient was also able to note that others had repeatedly told her she looked good in a short skirt, and that she felt she looked good as well. Subsequently the patient felt more confident about wearing short skirts.

After some weeks of addressing her body image concerns, another patient explained how a point that the therapist had discussed theoretically had recently become meaningful to her. She had noticed that there were some days when she "felt fat" but because she had been successfully maintaining her weight for several weeks she came to realize that objectively there had been no change in her physical state. She realized that the days when she "felt fat" were days that were particularly stressful or unpleasant, or times when she felt low in mood. It became clear to her that although she felt worse about her body on these days, changes in her shape and weight were not the cause.

Reality or Hypothesis Testing

Direct experiential testing is a powerful way of assessing the accuracy of negative predictions and of establishing and reinforcing alternative perspectives in the form of less self-critical thoughts and more functional beliefs. Such testing can help patients not just to see things differently but to actually experience them differently. The importance of such enactive procedures in achieving changes in the patient's mind-set has been emphasized by Teasdale (1997). Patients should be encouraged to devise ways of testing out their new views by planning, carrying out, and reviewing an agreed experiment.

A patient was about to be interviewed for an academic job. She was convinced that it would be impossible for her to perform well at the interview because, although she had achieved reasonable weight loss, she still regarded herself as unacceptably fat. She firmly believed that she would not be seriously considered for academic jobs, and this had resulted in previous poor performances at interviews. It became clear in discussion that during these interviews, she had been focusing on what the interviewers thought about her appearance rather than on telling them about her work.

To test the patient's view that she could not perform well because of her weight, the patient and therapist agreed to conduct an experiment to see whether she could improve her performance if she concentrated exclusively on communicating her interest and involvement in her work. It was explicitly acknowledged that she could not be certain that she would get the job, however well she performed, nor could she be certain that the people interviewing her would not be prejudiced against someone who was overweight. On the other hand she could find out whether she could perform well "despite" her weight. The patient and therapist used a role play to allow her to practice her new interview behavior.

As a result of this experiment, the patient discovered that it was possible to perform well despite her weight. Although she did not get the job, she was runner up and received positive feedback about her performance. More importantly she felt she had performed well, which was in marked contrast to her view about her previous performance at such interviews.

Another patient was troubled by the belief that her bottom was disproportionately large, and that this would be noticed by others.

The therapist devised a test of this belief with the patient in which she would try wearing a sweater that did not cover her bottom, and assess her level of discomfort and other people's responses. She found that far from getting negative comments, changing her style of dress elicited many compliments, particularly as different clothes enabled people to discern that she had lost weight.

The patient also agreed that as part of an attempt to tackle her assumptions about other people's views on the size her bottom (and the implications of that), she would ask a trusted friend for her opinion. She reported that she had an interesting conversation with her friend and had discovered two important things. First, her friend (whom she trusted to be totally honest) assured her that her bottom was not disproportionately large. Second, her friend confessed that she had always been concerned about a physical attribute of her own which she had never dared talk about. The patient was able to reassure her friend that in the 40 years of their friendship she had never even noticed the attribute that had so concerned her friend. This proved to be a very useful point to the patient as it illustrated clearly how something that one considers to be of great significance may never have attracted the attention of others. The patient continued to experiment with different styles and colors of clothes, and became much more confident about her appearance.

Considering the Advantages and Disadvantages of Particular Ways of Thinking

In addition to evaluating the evidence on which they are based, self-critical thoughts and dysfunctional beliefs may also be challenged by considering the effects they have on the individual's feelings and behavior. Patients should be encouraged to examine the advantages and disadvantages of their view with particular reference to the way they feel and behave as a result. The therapist should encourage patients to identify any possible disadvantages of their views and to explore alternative perspectives that may be more helpful.

A patient reported feeling very fat and frumpy at a party with work colleagues. She described thinking that everyone present was thinner and more attractive than she was, and that they were probably thinking how awful she looked. She then began to think that she would never look good and that there was no point in bothering to lose weight because she would always be fat and she should just accept it. These thoughts made it very difficult to concentrate when talking to people, and she began to think she had nothing to say to others. As a result she drank a great deal of alcohol to feel more confident and less miserable, and she also ate more than she had planned. In discussion with the therapist, the patient was able to see that thinking in the way she had at the party had resulted in her finding it more difficult to talk to people, and she had enjoyed the party less and eaten and drunk more than she had planned. She was also able to see that if she had concentrated on the fact that she had felt good when she dressed for the party, that she had received some compliments about her dress and that among the people present there were not only people who were thinner than she, but also some who were larger, she would have become involved in interesting conversations and enjoyed the party. Also she would have been more likely to stick to her plan for eating and drinking.

Identifying and Correcting Biased Perception and Interpretation

Patients should be helped to identify and correct the biases in their self-critical thoughts and dysfunctional beliefs. There are a number of common biases in the perception and interpretation of information. The main ones are listed below together with the means of addressing them.

Selective Attention.   Many patients with body image concerns show selective attention to information (events and experiences) that is consistent with their negative views of their bodies. Thus patients tend to focus only on what are viewed as negative aspects of appearance or only pay attention to and make comparisons with people who are thought to be thinner and more attractive than they are and never with those who may be larger and less attractive. To address selective attention, the therapist should first educate the patient about the phenomenon. In general people pay particular attention to stimuli that are highly personally salient. This can be illustrated with an example. Patients could be asked whether they have ever bought a new car. If so, did they suddenly start to notice many more cars like theirs? Patients will acknowledge that the number of these cars is unlikely to have changed, but because the car was on their mind and had special significance they were noticing similar cars. Examples of selective attention should be sought, ideally from the patients' own experience. The goal is to help patients realize that their body image concerns lead to such issues being highly salient to them, which in turn results in their paying particular attention to their concerns, which in turn maintains their dissatisfaction. Broadening the patient's focus of attention should therefore be a goal of treatment.

To address selective attention, identifying the situations in which it occurs is an essential first step. Simply noting down some such situations is helpful because they can be subsequently discussed in session. The therapist's goal is then to help the patient learn to broaden her or his attention *at the time* that the selective attention occurs. For example, patients who only notice their hips (which they dislike) should actively pay attention to other more neutral parts of their body such as their hair or eyes, whereas those who only notice others who are thinner than they are, should actively pay attention to those who are not thinner or even those who are larger.

Discounting Positive Aspects of Appearance.   Many patients with body image concerns notice and recall only negative events related to shape, weight, and appearance and overlook positive ones (or the absence of expected negative comments). Identifying positive events, such as being paid a compliment, can help patients achieve a more balanced appraisal of these matters. To do this, patients should note down anything positive that occurs with regard to their appearance, and they should actively look out for such events. The absence of any expected negative event should also be recorded (e.g., going to a party and not receiving negative comments on his or her appearance).

Double Standards.   Patients with body image concerns may have one set of (harsh) standards for judging their shape, and another (more lenient) set for others. They may also believe that others judge them by the same harsh standards they use for themselves. Addressing double standards primarily involves helping patients to recognize when they operate in this fashion, and then reviewing in detail any justification for such double standards. This should include a review of the justification for the belief that others, unlike the patient, apply the patient's harsh standards to everyone. Usually just highlighting the phenomenon is sufficient to erode it.

A patient who had lost more than 10% of her body weight remained very unhappy with her shape and wanted to lose more weight. When discussing the body image checklist, she mentioned that she avoided shopping for clothes and she also avoided wearing clothes that showed her shape. She reported that she felt ashamed of her body and thought that other people were critical about her because of her shape. She said that the clothes she had been wearing at the start of treatment did not feel any looser and that no one had commented on her weight loss.

The therapist suggested that people might be more likely to comment positively on her changed appearance if she tried wearing different clothes. The patient said she would think about getting new clothes, but seemed reluctant to do so.

At the following session, the patient said she had found a photograph of herself before she had started losing weight, and she was amazed at the change that she could see. She also reported that she had received some positive comments from other people about her weight loss. The therapist discussed selective attention with her, and the patient agreed that she had previously failed to take note of positive comments, and only remembered when people had not commented about her weight loss. As homework the therapist asked the patient to record any negative thoughts she had about her body during the next week.

At the following session, the patient described one example of a negative thought, when she had caught sight of herself in a shop window and had automatically thought, "You haven't lost weight at all." She had then challenged this thought and acknowledged that she *had* lost a significant amount of weight. She realized that she assumed that people were judging her negatively because that was the way that she judged herself. This was discussed at length during the session.

The next week the patient said that she was happy to accept her weight even if she did not lose any more weight. She reported that she had not had any more negative thoughts about her body. When she began the weight maintenance stage, she bought herself a new outfit, which she felt pleased to wear as evidence that she positively accepted her new shape. She stated that she had begun to wear short skirts and no longer dressed to disguise her shape.

Overgeneralization.   Patients with body image concerns may tend to equate not succeeding in achieving their weight and shape goals as evidence that they are a failure more generally. This is addressed in the same way as double standards. The therapist first helps patients identify the phenomenon when it occurs and then in-session asks patients to justify the basis for their thinking, the aim being to counter the phenomenon.

Dichotomous Thinking.   This is also common among patients with body image concerns (e.g., "I have not reached my ideal weight (thin) so I must be fat," "To be respected I must be thin."). These examples of black-and-white thinking can be addressed by reviewing evidence, reaching a balanced conclusion, and conducting an experiment to test out the new conclusion. Sometimes the use of adaptive and orthogonal continua (see Padesky, 1994) are useful to illustrate the nature of this thinking, as illustrated in the examples below.

A patient who had lost 10% of her body weight, but was still 11 lb (5 kg) from her ideal weight, continued to think of herself as fat and no different from before she had lost weight. The evidence she cited for this view was that she had not reached her ideal, which was the only weight at which she would see herself as not fat. This was proving an obstacle to her accepting her new weight and being prepared to maintain this weight. Instead she wished to lose further weight. The therapist discussed this issue and then drew a line (see Figure 7.2) to represent thinness (defined as being at ideal weight). One end was labeled as 0%, or

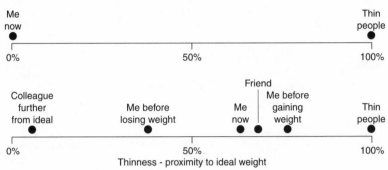

FIGURE 7.2 Adaptive continuum

not at ideal weight (fat), and the other end was labeled 100%, or at ideal weight. The patient was asked to locate herself and people who were thin on the line. She put herself at 0% (i.e., fat) and located thin people at 100%. The therapist then asked her whether it would be possible to be further from ideal weight than she was and whether she knew someone who was in this position. The patient volunteered that one of her work colleagues was further from ideal than she was, and so she was asked to put the colleague at the appropriate place on a new, similar line. The therapist asked her where she would put herself before her recent weight loss and also suggested that she mark the place where she would put a friend whom she thought did not look fat, but was not at her ideal weight. The patient also marked the place where she was before gaining weight when she had not thought she was fat. Finally the therapist asked her to locate herself on the new line. The therapist then helped her arrive at a new perspective. The patient concluded that although she had not reached her ideal weight, she weighed less than before and was thinner. She said further that she did not regard her friend as fat but her friend was nearly as far from her ideal as she was. Finally she concluded that it did not seem very accurate to regard someone who was not at their ideal weight as fat. This helped the patient to begin to accept her weight and agree to start weight maintenance.

Another patient was convinced that she would not be respected unless she was thin because she and others only respected thin people. The therapist drew two intersecting lines (see Figure 7.3), one indicating degrees of respect and the other thinness. The therapist and patient identified that the patient regarded the relationship between respect and thinness as linear (as shown on Figure 7.3) and then located a number

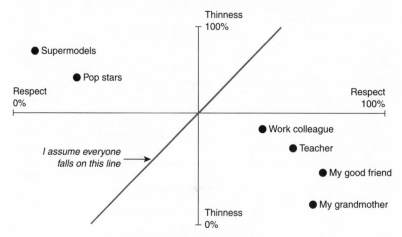

FIGURE 7.3 Orthogonal continuum

of people respected by the patient and others who did not fit onto this line. The patient was able to see that, in practice, both she and others respected people for reasons other than their weight, and this enabled her to make progress toward weight maintenance rather than trying to lose more weight.

When reviewing another patient's body image checklist, it became apparent that her negative thoughts about her body were contributing significantly to her problems. The patient described her thoughts and feelings about her body, and from this discussion the therapist and patient were able to distill several key thoughts. They noted these down, and the therapist asked the patient to consider these for homework to see if she could come up with any more neutral alternatives. Before the session ended, they discussed how the patient might go about this. The therapist recommended that the patient try asking herself questions such as: Is this statement objectively true? What is the evidence for it? What would I say to a friend who felt like this? Am I assuming what other people will think? Even if they were thinking those things, what difference would this really make—and what does it say about them?

The patient considered all this for homework and came back with a list of specific thoughts and alternative viewpoints:

They will think I cannot control my eating.

- They may not even think that, particularly if they do not see me with food. I probably would not think that of someone else.
- Do I really care if they do think that?

They will think that I overeat, and that is disgusting (and thus I am disgusting).

- Eating is not disgusting—it is necessary for life. I eat well and I do not overeat, so if they think I do it is their problem.
- Even if I do overeat, that does not make me disgusting.

I feel I must please everyone.

- Why? The most important person is actually me. It is good to be nice to others, but more important to be nice to oneself—and that means not torturing oneself.

They might think I am not perfect, and I count for nothing if I am not perfect.

- Yes, they might think that, but no one is perfect and everyone still counts. Being valuable is more important, and I will be more valuable if I am relaxed and accepting about my body and myself.
- People can and do tolerate the fact that everyone has a mix of different attributes and that nobody is perfect. People are still valued, despite imperfections.

They will see the fat and think it looks horrible. Then they will not respect me (professionally).

- People think different things about fat, so I cannot assume that people think it is horrible.
- Respect comes with what you do and who you are, not what you look like. I would respect someone regardless of their size.

The patient reported that she did not always fully believe her new alternative thoughts. The therapist reassured her this was normal and asked her to carry on "answering" (either in writing or mentally) any negative or biased thoughts that popped into her head. She did this, and over the course of the next 10 weeks became adept at doing it. These cognitive shifts helped her to try buying and wearing more closely fitting clothes, which served to further improve her body image.

Patients should be helped to identify the strategies that are most likely to be helpful under the circumstances. Then together the therapist and patient should identify, question, and address at least one or two thoughts in the session. It is helpful to write this process down in the body image diaries making full use of the "alternative thoughts" column. It is important in carrying out this process that the alternative thoughts or interpretations acknowledge the patient's concerns and the real situation, rather than becoming banal examples of "positive thinking" in which the patient does not believe. For example, alternatives would not necessarily be, "I look really good," but perhaps, "Although I weigh more than I would like to, I can still look stylish." Learning to challenge thoughts in this fashion takes several consecutive sessions. Therapists should be careful not to become didactic, trying to persuade the patient to change his or her beliefs, as this is often ineffective and may become little more than an argument. Rather, patients should be encouraged to look for alternatives themselves.

There is value in coming up with alternative views to problematic thoughts or attitudes, even if the patient does not fully believe the alternative. The simple process of questioning the initial thought or attitude can help patients to distance themselves from it and to hold it less firmly. It is also important to stress that such cognitive work should lead to experimenting with new perspectives and behavior (e.g., experimenting with different clothes, asking a friend's opinion, deciding to try out something that had previously been avoided). The results of such changes are likely to reinforce modifications in thoughts and attitudes.

Patients should also be asked to continue cognitive work as homework. They should be asked to write down in their body image diaries one or two examples that occur during the week, and also to record how they attempted to challenge them, and what the outcome was. This homework should then be reviewed in detail at the next session, and any difficulties explored. Therapists should always encourage and help patients to adopt a different perspective if appropriate. Such homework will generally need to be repeated over several sessions.

If patients appear to be so overwhelmed by their distress about their shape and weight that they have great difficulty completing relevant homework between sessions, then it may be preferable to perform this work within the session itself, as illustrated in the following vignette.

A patient who was very concerned about her body image had considerable difficulty completing homework assignments. It was therefore necessary to address her concerns without the benefit of body image diaries. The patient seemed so overwhelmed by her distress over her body that she found it difficult to focus her thoughts.

The therapist said, "Clearly this whole topic is very distressing to you. I think it might be most helpful if we thought about a specific time when you felt bad about your body—if we could work out what was going on there and then, we might be able to transfer this to other situations. Can you think of a time recently when you felt uncomfortable about your body?" The patient cited a recent trip abroad during which she had tried to buy new clothes. The therapist asked, "Can you think yourself back to the situation—can you recall one particular store? What were you looking at? Did you try anything on? What happened next? Did the shop assistants speak to you?"

Having established exactly what happened, the therapist then guided the patient to recollect first what she had been feeling at the time, and from there what thoughts had prompted these feelings.

This process enabled the therapist to discover that the patient had been guessing the assistants' thoughts. She had assumed that, because she was (in her opinion) unattractive, the assistants would look down on her. She also believed they would assume that she had less money to spend and that they would not be as helpful to her as they would be to a more attractive woman.

After some discussion the patient and therapist were able to reach the conclusion that although some of these assumptions might be true (possibly shop assistants may target those whom they assume will be high spenders), there was no way of knowing if this was the case, and it was not helpful to make these assumptions. Making such an assumption had probably led her to act in a more self-deprecating manner, which may well in turn have influenced the assistants' responses to her.

This use of targeted questioning provided the basis for setting up a behavioral experiment to help question some of her original assumptions.

Body Image Concerns and Weight-Independent Goals

Most patients who have reached this point in addressing their body image will have been working at the same time on their weight goals (see Chapter 8) and primary goals (see Chapter 9). It should therefore be clear what the patient hopes to achieve from weight loss. The distinction will also have been made between those goals that are truly dependent on weight or shape and those that are not. Below are some examples:

Weight/shape-dependent goals:
- Wearing certain clothes
- Participating in certain sports (e.g., horseback riding)

Weight/shape-independent goals:
- Being more confident socially
- Socializing more
- Paying more attention to appearance (e.g., hairstyle)
- Buying new clothes
- Engaging in certain sports (e.g., swimming)
- Forming relationships

All patients should be strongly encouraged to address their weight-independent goals because not doing so is likely to reinforce their negative attitude toward their appearance and weight (as they will be viewed as barriers to progress in other areas). As discussed in Chapter 9, the patient and therapist should plan ways of achieving these weight-independent goals, and the patient's progress in this regard should be regularly reviewed.

Positive Acceptance

The notion of acceptance and change may well have been introduced already, while addressing the patient's weight goals (see Chapter 8). Therapists should also introduce this notion in relation to body image and suggest that acceptance may be enhanced by identifying sources of positive body image experiences. The points to cover are as follows:

- The patient has been making major efforts to lose weight and has thereby already (in most cases) changed his or her appearance.
- The patient will also have made other changes that will result in a less negative body image than before (e.g., by addressing body avoidance, checking and negative thinking).
- Having made these important changes, the patient needs to learn to accept his or her body and weight, and in addition, accept the fact that, although he or she may desire further change, this may not be possible.
- So far acceptance has mainly involved encouraging patients to be less negative about their bodies than previously.
- It is possible for many patients to feel positive about their bodies by exploring a range of activities from which they derive pleasure and satisfaction (e.g., sporting activities such as walking or swimming, being fit, sex, buying attractive clothes, changing hairstyle, etc.).

The patient and therapist should work together to identify activities that might encourage more positive attitudes toward his or her body. Often it is helpful to look for activities that patients used to like (and perhaps were good at) but have subsequently abandoned. They should be encouraged to reengage in such activities. These should be carefully planned so as to ensure a positive outcome, and the patient's experience should be carefully reviewed. As before, it is helpful to ask patients to predict the outcome, and later to compare the actual outcome with the expected one. The positive aspects of such activities should always be stressed. If necessary, patients should be helped to reframe the outcome in positive terms. This process is likely to extend over several sessions. (If this process involves increasing physical activity, see the guidelines in Chapter 6.)

A patient who had lost a substantial amount of weight, but not as much as she had desired, described herself as accepting her new weight because she no longer "stood out in a crowd." Further discussion revealed that although she no longer had strong negative feelings about her body, she did not feel particularly positive either and for this reason was somewhat apprehensive about buying new clothes. Although she knew that she "would be no different from others," she had no confidence that she would look good. She agreed to find out and bought a skirt, which she felt looked good on her. This success gave her confidence to buy other clothes, as did the compliments she received.

CHAPTER 8

Module VI: Addressing Weight Goals

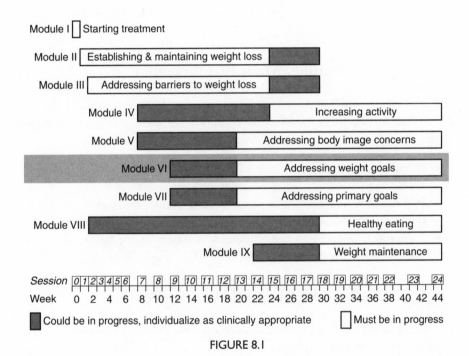

Module I ☐ Starting treatment

Module II | Establishing & maintaining weight loss |

Module III | Addressing barriers to weight loss |

Module IV | Increasing activity |

Module V | Addressing body image concerns |

Module VI | Addressing weight goals |

Module VII | Addressing primary goals |

Module VIII | Healthy eating |

Module IX | Weight maintenance |

Session 0 1 2 3 4 5 6 7 8 9 10 11 12 13 14 15 16 17 18 19 20 21 22 23 24
Week 0 2 4 6 8 10 12 14 16 18 20 22 24 26 28 30 32 34 36 38 40 42 44

■ Could be in progress, individualize as clinically appropriate   ☐ Must be in progress

FIGURE 8.1

One of the premises underlying this cognitive-behavioral treatment is that a major obstacle to successful weight maintenance is having an unrealistic goal when trying to lose weight. As explained in Chapter 2, this undermines the patient's ability to acquire and use effective weight maintenance behavior. The aim of this module is therefore to help the patient adopt and accept an appropriate goal weight. Achieving this goal involves the following specific steps:

1. Identifying weight goals.
2. Questioning the patient's "desired" weight.
3. Identifying primary (i.e., nonweight-related) goals.
4. Reviewing the causes of poor weight maintenance.
5. Identifying the benefits of moderate weight loss.
6. Emphasizing the need for "acceptance and change."
7. Encouraging acceptance.

A Note on Therapist Style

This module should take the form of a guided discussion, the intention being that the patients will reappraise their weight goals and, if appropriate, begin to adjust them. At the same time, therapists and patients should continue focusing on adherence to behaviors specified in Chapter 4 in order to achieve weight loss.

It generally takes at least three consecutive sessions to work through this module, and appropriate homework is needed after each session. The rate of progress varies markedly from patient to patient. It is important that the process is not hurried.

Determining When to Enter Module VI

This module should not be entered too early in treatment and weight loss should certainly be well established. We use the following guidelines (see Figure 8.1):

- It may be entered from week 12 if the patient is succeeding in steadily losing weight and is raising the topic of weight goals.
- It should be entered if, after a reasonable period of weight loss, the patient's weight loss is showing signs of tapering off for no obvious reason.
- It should be entered by the middle of treatment at the latest. (Our practice has been always to enter this module by week 20.)

Identifying Weight Goals

The therapist should initiate discussion of the patient's current weight goals by explaining that now that weight loss is underway, it is helpful to review in detail what the patient would like to achieve as a result of treatment. In practice most patients have a number of goal weights, although these are often not well formulated or differentiated. The therapist's first task is to help patients clarify them. Three goal weights should be distinguished, an ideal (or "dream") weight, a desired weight, and a tolerable weight. These may be defined as follows:

1. *Ideal weight.* This is the weight that patients would very much like to achieve although they appreciate that it is a dream weight that is unrealistic for them at this stage in their life. It should be a weight that they think they could conceivably reach, while knowing that doing so is extremely unlikely. They would not feel that treatment had failed should they not reach this weight.
2. *Desired weight.* This is the weight that patients think they should, and probably could, achieve during treatment. Objectively it may also be un-

realistically low, but it is nevertheless the goal they wish to achieve. They would think they (or the treatment) had failed if they did not reach this weight.

3. *Tolerable weight.* This is the highest goal weight that they think they could accept. They would be disappointed if they only reached this weight, but it is a weight that they think they could tolerate and come to accept.

The process of identifying and differentiating these goal weights is the first step in beginning to modify them. The most important one to be clear about is the desired weight. If the patient has changed her or his weight goals since being asked to identify these in session 0, it may be useful to discuss this change. Such changes can reflect the arbitrary nature of weight goals and the patient's flexibility.

Some patients say that they do not have a goal weight, but do have a goal clothing size. If this is the case, the whole topic of weight goals can be discussed in terms of clothing size rather than weight. If the patient has no goal in terms of weight or size, and claims that he or she will be pleased with whatever weight loss is achieved, there may be no need to cover most of the material in this module. However, it would still be advisable to discuss previous experience of weight loss and regain, and educate the patient about the reasons weight is so often regained, as well as introducing the principle of "acceptance and change," discusssed later in this chapter.

If, on the other hand, patients say that they have no particular goal weight but just want to lose "as much weight as possible," they should be encouraged to identify what they would consider to be ideal, desired, and tolerable weights, as defined above, to enable further discussion. Therapists should acknowledge that patients may find it difficult to specify these goal weights, and therapists should say that the precise number is not important. Patients should also be told that they will not be held to these goals, and they can change their minds, but identifying their goals will give the therapist a rough idea of what they might be aiming for at the moment.

Questioning the Desired Weight

The next step in modifying the patient's weight goals is to examine their origins. This takes a session or more with homework in between. The focus should be on the patient's desired weight. This process is likely to demonstrate its arbitrariness as well as begin to suggest that it is unlikely to be achievable. The session should be structured around the following patient-oriented discussion points:

1. *Origins of the desired weight.* The therapist should review the origins of the patient's desired weight. Possible reasons for adopting a particular weight might be recommendations of physicians or weight-loss groups, following

weight charts, wishing to once again attain the lowest weight achieved as a result of previous weight loss attempts, a belief that the particular weight is necessary in order to achieve a primary goal (see next section), or a variety of other reasons that make a specific weight personally significant.

2. *Other weight goals in the past.* The therapist should review previous attempts to lose weight and the patient's goals at the time.

3. *Achievability of the desired weight.* Prior attempts to maintain this weight or a weight near it should be reviewed. Also the patient should be asked whether they foresee any difficulties attempting to maintain it now.

4. *Importance of reaching the desired weight.* The personal importance attached to the attainment of the desired weight (i.e., what reaching this weight means to the patient) should be assessed.

5. *Consequences of reaching the desired weight.* Patients should be asked to consider how their lives would be different were they to reach this weight. For those who have previously achieved this weight, the discussion should focus on in what respects, if any, life was different.

When considering these issues it is useful to consider the following eight aspects of daily life:

- Attractiveness
- Clothing size and choice
- Health and fitness
- Leisure activities (e.g., sports)
- Work
- Social life
- Self-esteem and self-confidence
- Personal relationships

The therapist should review in detail each of these domains of functioning and the changes that the patient predicts would occur if he or she reached the desired weight. If applicable, it is helpful to refer back to times in the past when the patient was at this weight to see whether the patient's expectations are supported by past experience.

6. *Consequences of not reaching the desired weight.* The therapist should encourage the patient to consider how he or she would respond to not reaching the desired weight. It is important to assess how the patient would interpret not reaching this weight (i.e., their cognitive response) and their likely reaction to this interpretation (e.g., giving up attempts at weight control).

The patient handout "Your Weight Goals" (Handout R) lists a number of direct questions for the patient relating to these issues. It is often appropriate to cover items 1–4 in the session, and then discuss 5 and 6 in outline only and ask patients to consider them in more detail as homework (using the questions in the handout) and perhaps to write down their responses. At the end of the discussion the therapist should summarize the main points to establish whether the patient agrees with them. If there are any discrepancies, they should be explored and resolved.

Just before the halfway point in treatment, the therapist introduced the topic of weight goals. He explained to the patient that, as they would be spending approximately the last third of treatment practicing weight maintenance, it was important that they prepared themselves for this by reviewing her weight goals. The patient agreed to think about the questions on the "Your Weight Goals" handout for homework.

At the next session, the patient stated that she would like to start the weight maintenance phase at the following session. Having reviewed the questions on the handout, she decided that although in the long term she would like to lose some more weight, she would prefer to capitalize on what she had achieved so far by learning to maintain her weight and then consider further weight loss at some point in the future. The therapist explained that patients are encouraged to practice keeping their weight steady for at least 9 months before considering losing further weight. The patient said she was happy to do this. Although it was agreed that the patient would start the weight maintenance stage as she wished, the therapist nevertheless ensured that the relevant questions about weight goals were discussed. Although the patient had clearly reached the desired conclusion regarding the flexibility of weight goals, it remained important to identify and address her primary goals, and some of the questions from the weight goals handout were an important starting point for this discussion.

Identifying Primary Goals

In reviewing patient's weight goals and their beliefs about what they will gain as a result of weight loss, therapists should introduce the distinction between those goals that cannot be achieved without at least some weight loss (e.g., reduction in clothing size) and those that do not necessarily require weight loss (e.g., engaging in sports, feeling more self-confident). The latter may be described as "primary" goals.

Therapists should devote time to the identification of patient's primary goals. These should be real goals rather than flights of fantasy. They should be listed and patients should be encouraged to pursue those that could be achieved right away (e.g., taking up swimming, joining an evening class). In subsequent sessions therapists should routinely enquire about patients' progress toward these goals. Weight-dependent goals and those that are difficult to achieve should be put aside for the moment, although therapists should make it clear that they will be addressed later on. Goals related to body image should be addressed as described in Chapter 7.

A patient responded to the "Your Weight Goals" handout by listing a number of goals she hoped she would achieve by reaching her desired weight. These were: "to be able to go swimming; believe I can get another job (against a thin person); feel attractive, and feel it is worthwhile taking care of myself and my appearance." The patient and therapist reviewed this list to identify which of these goals were entirely weight dependent. The patient was able to see that none were strictly weight dependent and that it might be possible to achieve these goals without losing further weight. They also discussed her achievements to date (e.g., weight loss, improvements in confidence, etc.). The patient began to appreciate that, although she desired more weight loss, the changes that she had made so far were worthwhile in themselves.

The therapist also focused the discussion on the patient's belief that not achieving her goal weight would mean that she was useless and a failure. The patient followed this line of thinking in many aspects of her life—for example, believing she was a dreadful parent when one of her teenage sons got into trouble with the police. The therapist encouraged her to note down times when she felt she was a failure and to consider the evidence for and against these beliefs. It was recommended that she use questions such as "What would I think if one of my friends were in this situation?" to help her achieve a more objective viewpoint.

By the time the patient was due to embark on weight maintenance, she was happy to do so, and the therapist ensured that the work on achieving primary goals by means other than weight loss continued during this phase.

Another patient had got to within 7 lb (3.2 kg) of her desired weight by the time she was due to start weight maintenance. The therapist reviewed her primary goals with her in order to assess how much things would change if she did lose this extra weight. On doing so, the patient identified that she had either fully achieved, or made significant progress toward, most of her goals. She was doubtful as to how much more could be achieved by losing further weight. For example she felt that she had already improved her self-image to such an extent that she did not think that a further 7 lb would make a significant difference. She was able to identify that her main motivation for getting to the goal weight that she had identified at the start of treatment was to "see it through." She felt that she might see herself as a failure if she did not reach her goal (particularly as her mother had criticized her in childhood for not "seeing things through"). Further consideration of her primary goals enabled her to see that pursuing such an arbitrary goal was unlikely to have any benefit for her, and that she could find alternative ways to refute the critical voice of her mother.

Reviewing the Causes of Poor Weight Maintenance

This is an appropriate point in treatment to return to the principles of weight regulation (discussed in Chapter 4) so as to reinforce that information and stress that it is a skill that needs to be learned and practiced. The information provided should be kept simple and to the point. The points are covered in Table 4.3 (Handout E).

The aim of this discussion is to remind patients that limiting their food intake is hard work and that it would be asking too much of them to attempt to maintain indefinitely their present level of food restriction. Indeed, doing this would be setting themselves up to fail as the research evidence indicates that people find it increasingly hard to keep to a 1,200- to 1,500-calorie limit after 4–6 months, however successful they have been up to that point (see Wadden, Sarwer, & Berkowitz, 1999; Wilson & Brownell, 2002). Therapists should explain that a time will come when it will be clear that it would be better if patients stopped trying to lose weight and instead focused on learning how to maintain their new weight.

Experience of Weight Maintenance in the Past

While patients are still losing weight, therapists should initiate a discussion about the patient's previous experiences of weight loss and weight regain. The aim of this discussion is to help patients identify personally relevant factors that may have contributed to poor weight maintenance in the past. Most patients will have lost weight in the past and will have subsequently regained it. In such cases therapists should obtain a detailed account of what happened. It is best if the therapist starts by focusing on a recent (and representative) episode of weight loss and regain. The key points may be elicited by asking about the topics listed below. Only the most pertinent of these questions need to be asked. (It is not possible to do this with the few patients who have not attempted to lose weight in the past. Instead they should simply have the common sequence of events described to them in a way that invites them to speculate on what commonly happens at each point).

The weight loss phase

- Starting weight
- Amount lost
- Time taken to lose weight
- Match or mismatch between goals and what was achieved
- Patient's views about achievement or lack of it

Attempts at weight maintenance

- Reasons for stopping further attempts at weight loss: decision or gradual slowing down
- Decisions to maintain weight

For those who decided to try to maintain their new, lower weight

- Details of how the patient tried to maintain weight
- Knowledge about how to maintain weight
- Any help or advice from others
- Details of patient's eating: quantities eaten, type of food, etc.
- Details of weight monitoring, if any

For those who did not decide to maintain their new, lower weight

- Reasons for not deciding to maintain
- Views about new weight as compared to previous weight

Subsequent events

- Course of subsequent weight gain
- Reactions to regaining weight

For those who tried to counter the weight regain

- Details of attempts to reverse weight regain
- Reasons for abandoning weight control efforts, if applicable

For those who did not try to counter the weight regain

- Reasons for not trying to reverse the weight gain
- Acceptance of new lower weight (even if higher than desired)

For those who did not accept their new, lower weight

- Reasons for not accepting new weight
- Any perceived changes at new weight

The goal of this detailed questioning is to identify the relative contributions of the three mechanisms commonly responsible for poor weight maintenance:

1. *Having an unrealistic weight goal.* Failing to achieve their goal often results in patients' not attempting to maintain their new, lower weight or only attempting to do so in a half-hearted fashion. This is because they tend to see the weight loss they have achieved as paltry and therefore not worth maintaining (an example of dichotomous thinking).

2. *Having to maintain extreme dietary restraint in the long term.* If the patient needs to exert extreme dietary restraint in order to maintain the new, lower weight, weight regain is likely to occur because it is difficult for most patients to maintain high levels of restraint indefinitely. This vulnerability is often compounded by the abandonment of weight control efforts at any sign of weight regain (also an example of dichotomous thinking).

3. *Not knowing what is involved in successful weight maintenance.* Some patients do not realize that weight maintenance is an active process that requires thought and practice with adjustments being made in eating (and activ-

ity levels) in relation to changes in weight so that weight stabilization can be achieved and maintained.

Therapists should discuss the relative contributions of these mechanisms with the patient with the aim of collaboratively arriving at an individualized account (formulation) of why the patient failed to maintain the weight lost in the past. It may be helpful to use a simplified version of the cognitive account of weight maintenance (see Chapter 2), which stresses the contribution of two fundamental factors: inappropriate weight goals (the basis for explanations 1 and 2 on the previous page) and the lack of appreciation of what is involved in successful long-term weight maintenance.

Therapists can then explain how this treatment is designed to overcome these common problems by helping to establish appropriate weight goals and by providing the opportunity to acquire and practice weight maintenance skills. If the patient has regained weight many times in the past, it is especially important that the therapist appears encouraging and optimistic in describing how the outcome can be different this time.

A patient and therapist reviewed the patient's previous weight loss attempts. The patient described her last attempt when she had reached her desired weight but then had gradually regained the lost weight. She recalled that when she stopped going to her weight loss group, she drifted back to her former eating habits. She also noted that major life events had deflected her focus away from weight control. The therapist and patient concluded that weight regain was a result of not having established fundamental changes to her eating habits and not being aware of the need to approach weight maintenance proactively as a life-long endeavor.

Another patient recollected that she had maintained a lower weight the previous summer by sticking to an arduous regimen that involved doing a large amount of exercise and eating in a Spartan fashion on weekdays. She more or less abandoned these activities on the weekends. After some months she gave up trying and regained the lost weight. The patient and therapist concluded that having to stick to such a taxing regimen, plus not having worked out a way of including some "luxuries" without totally abandoning control was why she had not been able to maintain her new lower weight.

When asked about prior experience of weight loss and weight maintenance, a patient explained that when she had attended a commercial weight loss club, she had lost enthusiasm because she did not reach her goal weight. She had stopped weighing herself because she had "felt like a failure." She felt that it was not worth maintaining her new weight as she did not reach her goal, and she rapidly regained the lost weight. She said that this had been a common pattern in the past. On the occasion when she did reach her goal weight, she had to "starve herself" to maintain this weight. The patient and therapist identified her unrealistic weight goal and her "black-and-white" thinking pattern as contributing to a cycle of starving herself and overeating, and then, eventually, to her giving up and regaining the weight that she had lost.

The information on weight regulation, and the consideration of what happened in the past, leads naturally to a reevaluation of the patient's current desired weight. The issue of how to maintain weight can be put aside until weight loss begins to decrease (see Chapter 11).

In the light of these discussions, it may be useful to suggest that as homework the patient should list both the short-term and long-term pros and cons of their current desired weight. If the patient does not have a goal weight, he or she should be asked to list the pros and cons of losing more weight.

At assessment, a patient said that her desired weight was 154 lb (70.3 kg). This was the lowest weight she had been as an adult, and she believed that at this weight she could wear whatever she wanted. She said that she could tolerate being 172 lb (78.0 kg), but no higher.

During the course of treatment, she managed to lose weight steadily. At week 23, the therapist raised the issue of weight goals again. The patient said that her "dream" weight was still 154 lb (70.3 kg), but that her desired weight was anywhere between 154 and 172 lb (70.3–78.0 kg). This acceptance of a weight range appeared to be an example of her modifying her dichotomous thinking style. She no longer spoke of 172 lb (78.0 kg) as a "just tolerable" weight, but instead said that such a weight would be very acceptable for her, as she had been that weight when she got married and she had felt comfortable then and had been able to wear fashionable clothes. She believed that she would be able to wear a bikini and engage in water sports at this weight without feeling too self-conscious. She now considered 182 lb (82.5 kg) to be the highest weight that she could tolerate.

The therapist asked the patient to complete questions 5 and 6 from the "Your Weight Goals" handout as homework—considering how her life would differ if she reached her desired weight as compared to not reaching it. She produced detailed answers to the homework questions in which she explained that she was already experiencing substantial benefits from her weight loss. Nevertheless, she thought that if she reached her desired weight, she would not have to be so careful about "covering up," exercise would be easier, she would buy nicer clothes, her husband would find her more attractive, and she would feel a sense of achievement. If she did not achieve her weight goal, she wrote, "I would feel pleased to have lost as much weight as I have, but I would regret missing such a good opportunity to reach my desired weight. Weight maintenance might be more difficult. I would feel I had failed. . . . I also would not feel slim enough if I did not get to 172 lb (78.0 kg)."

In the following session, the therapist asked the patient about her prior experience of weight loss and weight maintenance. The patient explained that when she had attended a commercial weight loss club, she had "felt a failure" because she had not reached the goal weight of 147 lb (66.7 kg) she had been set, and she rapidly regained the lost weight. The one time she did reach 154 lb (70.3 kg), the goal she had wanted to achieve at the beginning of treatment, she had to "starve herself" to maintain this weight.

As the therapist and patient discussed her weight goals, the patient came to agree that her most important aim was to maintain the weight she had lost, even if she did not reach as low a weight goal as she was hoping for. She decided that the number on the scales was "not magical." The therapist then introduced the notion of acceptance and change. The patient reported that having lost 31 lb (14 kg), she already felt much better about herself and had more of a spring in her step. She said that she liked to look "curvy" (rather than like a "super-model"). She added that she felt she would be able to accept her maintenance weight, even if it was not as low as she had originally hoped for.

During this period of treatment, she continued to take steps to meet her "primary goals," which had been discussed at earlier sessions. She tried wearing tops that showed her tanned stomach instead of "covering up," and she received positive feedback from her family and friends. She continued to swim and cycle.

At week 32 the patient entered the weight maintenance stage of treatment, weighing 182 lb (82.5 kg). Although she had originally stated that she would not find this weight tolerable, she now said that she could happily accept this weight, and work to maintain it. Rather than feeling a failure, she said that she knew she had achieved a great deal by losing so much weight. She reported that she felt pretty positive about her appearance.

Identifying the Benefits of Moderate Weight Loss

The therapist should introduce the topic of the benefits of moderate weight loss by saying now that the patient is losing weight, it is time to consider the benefits such weight loss brings. Patients should be asked to think carefully about any positive changes that have already occurred. Their attention should be drawn to possible areas in which they may have experienced benefits—for instance, their level of energy, sense of well-being, fitness, mobility, ease of daily life, job performance, and so on. These should be discussed in some detail and, if necessary, therapists should help patients reframe what has been achieved in more positive terms. Therapists should encourage patients to see that, by recognizing their achievements, they are more likely to continue being successful. This can usually be done by drawing on the patient's experience of times in the past when success has led to an upward spiral of improved self-confidence and further success, and in contrast, times when perceived failure led to a downward spiral of poor self-confidence and further difficulties.

Therapists should supplement the review of benefits already achieved by presenting the following information about the health benefits of moderate weight loss. The benefits of 10–15% weight loss include the following:

- Improved appearance and decrease in waist size (and therefore clothing size)
  [If applicable, refer to any such changes reported to date.]
- Enhanced sense of general well-being and self-esteem
  [Refer to the fact that many people gain in self-respect, become more self-confident, and start doing things that they have been putting off for years. If applicable, refer to any such changes reported to date.]
- Decrease in many of the negative effects on health associated with obesity (e.g., high blood pressure, high blood lipids, high blood sugar) as well as the risk of developing these problems
  [Discuss with reference to the patient's current physical health.]
- Improved sense of physical well-being
  [Refer to many people feeling healthier—having more energy and feeling less physically tired—and to their taking up of new activities. If applicable, refer to any increases in physical well-being reported to date.]

As homework it is often appropriate to ask patients to list the benefits they have already obtained. In reviewing this homework, therapists should ensure that patients do not dismiss their achievements as insignificant.

Emphasizing the Need for Acceptance and Change

The next step is central to this form of treatment. It involves conveying to the patient the need for both acceptance and change. To successfully overcome the problem of obesity, patients need to change what can be changed, taking a long-term perspective, and to accept what cannot be changed (see Wilson, 1996). The points to stress (many of which have been referred to before) are listed below. Therapists should discuss each point in detail and reinforce the information by giving patients Handout S ("Acceptance and Change").[1]

This process should not be hurried and a collaborative questioning style should continue to be used with reference being made to the patient's own personal experiences and circumstances. It is helpful to give patients the handout to take away, and to ask them to reread it and bring any questions or comments back to the next session. The points to cover are as follows:

- Some aspects of the problem of being overweight can be changed; some cannot.
- A good treatment should help people change what can be changed and accept what cannot. An analogy may be drawn with diabetes mellitus. People with diabetes can learn what and when to eat and when to take insulin to reduce their risk of developing health problems, but they have to accept that they have diabetes and that the treatment does not remove the underlying medical condition. Likewise, people vulnerable to obesity can learn how to eat and exercise so that they keep the obesity "at bay" and remain healthy, but the underlying predisposition will remain.
- Body weight is, to an important extent, genetically determined and is therefore only partially under one's control.
- It is possible to make fairly dramatic short-term changes in weight by severely cutting down energy intake, but a great deal of research has shown that such changes can rarely be sustained in the long term.
- There is currently no treatment for obesity (other than gastrointestinal surgery) that results in a weight loss of more than 10–15% of initial body weight, and the weight lost is generally regained. Typically a third of the lost weight is regained within 1 year and almost all of it is regained within 5 years (see Wadden, Sarwer, & Berkowitz, 1999; Wilson & Brownell, 2002). This is true of all nonsurgical treatments (dietary treatments, very low calorie diets, behavior modification, and appetite suppressant drugs) as well as combinations of these treatments.
    [The therapist should work out what a 10–15% weight loss would represent for the patient and inform the patient.]
- Most people have a desired weight that is far lower than 10–15% weight loss.
    [The patient's desired weight should be compared with the 10–15% weight loss range.]
- As a result, people who try to lose more than this view treatment (or themselves) as having failed, whereas it is really an achievement to lose this amount of weight and keep it off.

---

[1] With patients who have lost less than 5% of their initial body weight, the slightly modified handout, Handout T, should be used instead.

- A weight loss of 10–15% has many benefits.

    [The therapist should list with the patient any benefits that they have experienced, for instance:

    - improved appearance and decrease in waist size (and therefore clothing size),
    - enhanced sense of general well-being and self-esteem,
    - decrease in many of the negative effects on health associated with obesity, as well as the risks of developing these problems, and
    - improved sense of physical well-being.]

- Simultaneous with weight loss, treatment can address other personal goals, and generally this has a very positive effect on quality of life.

    [The therapist should refer to patients' specific primary goals, highlight progress in this regard, and remind them that these goals will soon become a focus of treatment.]

The therapist should summarize by stressing the main implications of this information for the patient; namely:

- Patients can change their weight to an important extent (say 10% weight loss), although the weight loss may well not be as great as they would wish.
- They can directly address other important (primary) goals, but it is essential that they accept what cannot be changed (weight range, overall shape).
- If they do not succeed in accepting what cannot be changed, they are going to be at risk of:
    - undervaluing what has been achieved in treatment,
    - believing that weight cannot be controlled at all, and
    - not being fully committed to keeping off the weight that has been lost. In our experience, this is a major cause of weight regain. If applicable, this point should be stressed with reference to the patient's prior experience.

Appropriate homework involves asking patients to review their current desired weight and consider whether it needs to be adjusted upward. They should consider what the problems would be (if any) if they had a higher desired weight. Their conclusions should be reviewed in the next session with the aim of identifying obstacles to their acceptance of a more moderate weight goal. The aim is not to achieve a radical reappraisal of their weight goals, but rather to encourage a more flexible and pragmatic attitude with unrealistic and rigidly held goals being replaced, not by passive resignation, but rather by positive acceptance (Wilson, 1996).

A patient accepted that she would enter the maintenance phase of treatment in 6 weeks but stated that she would like to try to lose another 7 lb (3.2 kg) before doing so. She had a vacation coming up, and she wanted to feel more comfortable about wearing shorts and a swimming suit. The therapist was aware that the patient had lost less weight than this up to this point in treatment (week 24), and it was therefore unlikely that she would lose this amount in the next 6 weeks. Although the therapist did not wish to discourage further attempts at weight loss, she did not want to reinforce the patient's unrealistic goals.

The therapist responded along these lines: "If you are eager to lose some more weight, that's great. Let's talk about exactly what you would need to do to get your weight going down again. Then how about seeing how you progress over the next few weeks? As you know, your weight loss so far has been fairly slow, so setting yourself an overambitious goal just now would probably not be helpful. We also need to spend some time thinking about weight maintenance, and what that will involve. At some point soon you will need to switch from actively trying to lose weight to actively maintaining your current weight." Thus, in addition to helping the patient with her goal of weight loss, the therapist addressed the theme of acceptance.

The patient expressed some doubt about whether she would have a good vacation if she did not lose this amount of weight. The therapist responded by questioning this belief and suggested that they talk more about how the patient might enjoy her trip regardless of whether she lost a bit more weight.

In this way the therapist acknowledged the patient's wish to lose more weight without getting sidetracked into a discussion of specific goals and was also able to introduce one of the key concepts of weight maintenance in a way that was tailored to the patient's current concerns.

Encouraging Acceptance

Therapists should try to identify obstacles to patients' acceptance of more moderate weight goals. The main obstacles generally belong to the following categories:

- *Difficulty accepting that their weight goal may be unrealistic.* This cognitive shift may take some time to occur. It is generally assisted by the decline in the rate of weight loss that usually occurs after some months in treatment.
- *Difficulty seeing that the achievement of more modest weight loss is a "success."* In this regard, patients should be helped to consider what really constitutes success. They should be encouraged to consider the advantages and disadvantages of briefly reaching a weight that is difficult to maintain and then regaining the weight lost, as compared to a more modest, but maintained, reduction in weight coupled with the tackling of the

patient's primary goals. Even if the patient has not lost weight, putting a stop to gradual weight gain should itself be seen as a success.

Although a patient had been having difficulty giving treatment priority in her life (in terms of attendance and homework), when weight goals were discussed, it became clear that her goals were still overambitious. After 18 weeks of treatment her weight was less than 2 lb (0.9 kg) below her initial weight, but she felt strongly that failing to lose 44 lb (20 kg) would indicate dreadful personal failure. Clearly, achieving such a weight loss in the remaining period of treatment would be impossible. The therapist was aware that unless the patient reached some acceptance of her current weight, she would be at high risk for abandoning her weight control attempts altogether—which would probably result in weight gain.

The patient's attendance continued to be poor. This meant that only three more sessions were held before the end of treatment, and so little time was available. However, the patient did become more accepting of weight maintenance during this time, acknowledging that she had been trying to lose weight during an exceptionally busy period in her life. She started to see her modest weight loss less as a personal failure and more as a product of circumstance, and she agreed that it was important, and an achievement at that point in her life, to maintain a stable weight.

- *Lack of progress in tackling primary goals and body image concerns.* Both are important. The distinction between weight-related and primary goals should be maintained. The patient's primary goals should become a focus of each session (see Chapter 9). As already discussed, body image concerns are addressed in Chapter 7.

During the transition between addressing weight goals and the starting of weight maintenance, the therapist asked the patient to consider what (if any) barriers remained to her acceptance of a higher weight than she had initially hoped for. The patient decided that her negative body image was the only significant problem. The patient and therapist decided that it would be helpful if the patient started maintenance at the agreed time, while also addressing her concerns about body image.

- *Wanting to achieve a specific goal weight, often defined as being below a certain "magic" number.* Some patients have a fixed goal weight that they wish to achieve (e.g., to be 175 lb; or to be less than 150 lb). It should be pointed out that such numbers are often arbitrary in nature—for example, depending on whether the patient thinks in kilograms or pounds, they are likely to select different goals. Therapists should point out the importance of accepting the achievement involved in the weight already lost rather than trying to reach a specific "goal weight."

A patient expressed the desire to achieve a certain weight by the time she started weight maintenance. The therapist questioned the patient further about this. Why would 175 lb (79.4 kg) be acceptable, but above this not? The patient thought about this, and was able to appreciate that this was an example of "black-and-white" thinking. After some discussion it was agreed that the patient should not pin all her hopes on achieving a specific weight. The patient could see that viewing 175 lb as acceptable but 176 lb as awful was not rational.

In fact, by the time weight maintenance started, the patient had reached 176 lb (79.8 kg). She did not interpret this as disastrous, and as maintenance progressed she became more comfortable with the idea that her weight would naturally fluctuate within a range. The important thing for her was to appreciate the many benefits she had gained from her weight loss and her new more relaxed eating style, rather than being unduly focused on her actual weight.

- *Wishing to continue losing weight, rather than accepting the weight already reached.* Under such circumstances the therapist should review the rationale for learning weight maintenance skills while still in treatment.

Patients may understand the rationale for moving on to weight maintenance, and may appear to "accept" their current weight in an intellectual sense but not really believe it enough to act accordingly. In one case a patient phrased it thus: "I can see it logically, but I do not believe it" (that it would be best to stop losing weight and practice weight maintenance instead). Another patient said, "I would rather lose more weight, but as everything else you have said so far has been true, I am willing to go along with you on this." In both cases the therapist was able to reassure the patient that it is normal to have doubts about acting in accordance with a new perspective of this type, however rational it might seem. In these circumstances, the therapist should suggest that patients experiment with the new perspective by acting as if they really believed it and note the results.

CHAPTER 9

Module VII: Addressing Primary Goals

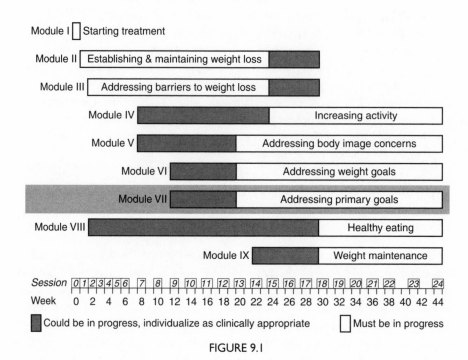

Module I ☐ Starting treatment

Module II | Establishing & maintaining weight loss |

Module III | Addressing barriers to weight loss |

Module IV | Increasing activity |

Module V | Addressing body image concerns |

Module VI | Addressing weight goals |

Module VII | Addressing primary goals |

Module VIII | Healthy eating |

Module IX | Weight maintenance |

Session 0 1 2 3 4 5 6 7 8 9 10 11 12 13 14 15 16 17 18 19 20 21 22 23 24
Week 0 2 4 6 8 10 12 14 16 18 20 22 24 26 28 30 32 34 36 38 40 42 44

■ Could be in progress, individualize as clinically appropriate   ☐ Must be in progress

FIGURE 9.1

Primary goals are objectives, other than weight loss, that patients are hoping to achieve as a result of losing weight. Few patients are exclusively interested in weight loss per se (i.e., the number on the weighing scale); rather, weight loss is a means to other ends. Among the many such primary goals are changes in appearance, enhanced fitness, better health, and greater self-confidence. The goals of this module are as follows:

1. To identify primary goals.
2. To address these goals.
3. To provide a more detailed description of some of the more common primary goals that patients may have.

Addressing the patient's primary goals is an important part of this cognitive-behavioral treatment. If weight loss is the sole focus of treatment, important additional goals may not be successfully met, with the result that, even if the goal weight is reached, certain aspects of the problem that led the patient to seek treatment may not have been overcome. This puts patients at risk of making further attempts at weight loss, which may, in turn, undermine successful weight maintenance. Conversely, successfully addressing patients' primary goals is likely to result in greater satisfaction with any weight loss achieved (even if it is not as much weight as they had originally hoped). As suggested earlier, greater satisfaction with what is achieved in treatment is likely to lead to better long-term weight maintenance.

It is therefore important that patients realize that many goals may be tackled and achieved independently of weight loss.

General Strategy for Tackling Primary Goals

Identifying Primary Goals

The patient's various goals for treatment will have been discussed in outline as part of the initial assessment process (see Chapter 3). The therapist does not need to delineate the full range of the patient's primary goals until weight goals become the focus of treatment (see Chapter 8). In practice, it is not uncommon for some primary goals to emerge earlier on in treatment, and if the patient is able to begin addressing them without being distracted from the priority of establishing and maintaining weight loss, this should be encouraged. On the other hand, if the patient is finding it difficult to lose weight, it is generally best if the therapist explains that it is not necessary for such additional goals to be tackled just yet (see Figure 9.1).

Addressing primary goals needs to be dovetailed with addressing body weight. The first step is to identify and distinguish the patient's various primary goals. Often there are several interrelated goals; for example, to become fitter and healthier. Some goals are weight dependent and therefore necessitate weight loss (e.g., to decrease clothing size); but many others are not directly weight related (for example, to have a better social life). The latter class of goal has the potential to be addressed independently of weight loss.

Addressing Primary Goals

Once the patient's various primary goals have been defined, they should each be addressed using the problem-solving approach described in Chapter 4. This involves identifying a wide range of potential solutions for each problem, selecting the most appropriate, implementing them, and then evaluating the chosen solution. This will generally involve both a long-term plan and specific short-term tasks that will take the form of homework. For example, a lonely patient who wants to have a better social life might decide to join a walking club as a short-term experiment. Joining the club and subsequent attendance at its meetings would become a regular item on the agenda of the treatment sessions. It might lead on to other social possibilities, which in turn would become the focus of sessions and the subject of problem solving. It must be noted, however, that primary goals should rarely be the main item on the agenda, and they should never take precedence over the achievement of weight loss and maintenance. On the other hand, they should not be forgotten.

Patients need encouragement and support to identify and tackle weight-independent primary goals while they are addressing their weight. Work on other weight-dependent goals has to wait until the necessary weight loss has been achieved. Often progress in tackling primary goals facilitates efforts at both weight loss and weight maintenance.

A patient held the view that she could not take swimming lessons until she reached her target weight. However, by the time the weight maintenance phase of treatment was close, it was apparent that she would still be at least 14 lb (6.3 kg) above her target weight. On asking the patient which of her goals were weight dependent and which were not, the patient was clear that taking swimming lessons was not really weight dependent. The therapist therefore asked her, as homework, to consider what it was that was stopping her going swimming. At the next session the patient explained that she believed that others would look at her in her swimming suit and view her as fat, and that believing this is how others would see her made her feel very uncomfortable. She went on to acknowledge that she had no evidence for this. Indeed she realized on reflection that the others in the beginners class were more likely to be preoccupied with their survival rather than the shape of their fellow learners. She also remembered that she had seen swimming suits in shops in sizes much larger than hers, and therefore felt that she was unlikely to be particularly noticeable.

The therapist praised the patient for thinking this through so carefully, and encouraged her to take another step toward fulfilling her goal by finding out about swimming classes in her area.

Common Primary Goals

To Improve Physical Appearance

The goal of improving physical appearance (i.e., the whole figure or aspects of it) may be motivated by patients' wishing to look better for their own sake or by a desire to be more physically attractive to others. Losing weight generally increases satisfaction with physical appearance, although this does not always happen. On the other hand, patients can become more accepting of their shape irrespective of the degree of weight loss. Some patients agree that the problem is not so much their weight (the number on the scale), but what they think about their weight. Therefore, losing weight is not the only solution; another solution is to address their attitude to their weight (see Chapter 7). Patients should also be reminded that people of any weight can make themselves look more attractive, and just because someone's weight is high does not necessarily mean that they are unattractive. Patients should be encouraged to do things that help them feel better about their appearance (e.g., wear different clothes, change their hairstyle or use make-up; see below).

To Increase Choice of Clothes

This is a common goal. It usually stems from a desire to look more attractive in general. Weight loss can increase the patient's options with regard to type and availability of clothes. During treatment, many patients have a tendency to delay buying new clothes in the hope that they will lose further weight and be able to fit into a smaller clothing size. Therapists should counter this by encouraging patients to buy new clothes in the course of losing weight. This is good for patients' morale and can have positive secondary effects (e.g., eliciting compliments from others). Similar considerations apply to changing other aspects of appearance (e.g., hairstyle and make-up). It is especially important for patients in the weight maintenance phase of treatment to have clothes appropriate to the size that they are learning to maintain—indeed, this is a good index of their degree of "acceptance." Dealing with avoidance of certain types of clothes is discussed in Chapter 7.

To Be Healthier

This is a major concern of some patients, particularly those who have developed weight-related medical problems such as hypertension, Type II diabetes, or problems with weight-bearing joints. It is also common among those with a family history of weight-related health problems (e.g., cardiovascular disease). In the main this primary goal need not be directly addressed because the changes in food choice, activity level, and weight loss that are integral to the treatment have important positive effects on health. It is now reasonably well established that even moderate weight loss (5–10% of initial body weight) has important health benefits, even if the patient remains significantly overweight (see Blackburn, 2002). For patients who have been steadily gaining weight, stopping this weight gain reduces their health risks, even if no weight is lost. Patients should have been informed about this already (see Chapters 3 and 8), and should be reminded if necessary.

To Be Fitter

Some patients are concerned about their level of fitness. This may stem from difficulty engaging in everyday activities (e.g., playing with children, walking up hills, climbing stairs, etc.) or it may arise from a desire to take up a sport or physically active pastime. All patients should be encouraged to be more physically active as part of a permanent lifestyle change. This is integral to the treatment and is addressed in Chapter 6. Often becoming fitter has valuable secondary effects; for example, it commonly improves self-respect and body image, and, in the case of sports that involve others, it may have valuable interpersonal benefits.

To Have Better Relationships

Ways of establishing a more rewarding interpersonal life can only be addressed to a degree in the context of this treatment. The comprehensive tackling of longstanding interpersonal deficits is outside the scope of this treatment. Patients should certainly be encouraged to be socially more active, and they should be supported in their efforts in this regard. Like buying new clothes, making changes in this domain should not be delayed until a specific weight is reached. Patients should be encouraged to set small, specific goals. Should they not manage to meet their goal, they should use problem solving to identify the obstacles, and if necessary, set a new, less demanding goal.

To Have More Self-Respect and Self-Confidence

These are complex goals. Problems with self-respect and self-confidence may range in severity from some degree of demoralization (perhaps as a result of weight gain) in a person with reasonable prior self-esteem to severe, chronic, and global negative self-evaluation. Treatment generally results in improved self-respect and self-confidence, especially in those patients with less severe problems in this area. In particular, the enhanced control over eating (especially in those who used to binge eat), the weight loss, the increase in activity level, and the greater acceptance of shape and weight contribute to improved self-evaluation. In addition, general cognitive work on dichotomous reasoning and negative thinking is often successful in helping patients to evaluate themselves in a more balanced way. On the other hand, such changes and procedures tend to have limited effect in those patients with more severe and longstanding low self-esteem. Addressing the negative self-concept of these patients is beyond the scope of this treatment.

Just as with other weight-independent goals, patients who want to lose weight to improve their self-confidence should be encouraged to consider whether there are other means by which they could increase their confidence. They should be encouraged to explore a range of options and then take steps to experiment with those possibilities that they think are most likely to help to improve their confidence.

To Make Life Changes

Some patients have plans to change aspects of their life once they have lost weight. Often these changes have been put "on hold" until the weight loss is achieved. Examples include changing jobs, taking up a new pastime, and leaving an unsatisfactory relationship. In general therapists should encourage patients to work toward such goals so long as doing so is not likely to interfere with weight loss and weight maintenance.

Discussion of primary goals can lead to the realization that particular goals cannot be achieved by weight loss per se and may indeed be outside the scope of this treatment.

A patient who had hoped that weight loss might improve her marriage, came to realize that her husband did not notice her weight—whether high or low—and that weight loss was therefore unlikely to affect the relationship. The therapist made it clear that there are certain things that cannot be dealt with in the course of weight control treatment, telling the patient, "I am happy to help you in every way I can to lose weight, but it is important that we recognize that doing so may not sort out the problems within your marriage. On the other hand, losing weight is an important thing you can do for yourself, and it can still have great benefits to you personally."

In some cases patients may not pursue their primary goals, even when they have reached their target weight or have come to recognize that the goal is not dependent on weight loss. There may be other barriers to achieving these goals, such as money or time, and not achieving them does not necessarily constitute a failure of treatment. Most important is that patients recognize that it is not their weight alone that is holding them back from achieving their goals, as believing that weight is the only barrier tends to encourage patients to have a negative view of their weight and shape and to attempt to lose further weight.

A therapist asked a patient to list her primary goals as homework and to assess which of them could only be achieved through weight loss and which were not weight-dependent.

The patient listed as her primary goals: (1) to improve choice in clothes, (2) to increase confidence/decrease feelings of being conspicuous, (3) to be able to go swimming.

The patient reported that she had figured out that none of her goals were absolutely weight dependent. She believed that she could try some new clothing stores and also increase her level of exercise (including going swimming), both of which would increase her self-confidence. The therapist and patient were then able to work on developing the patient's exercise program. They were also able to investigate other ways of helping the patient achieve her primary goals—for example, addressing the biased thoughts that made her feel conspicuous, particularly at the swimming pool.

CHAPTER 10

Module VIII: Healthy Eating

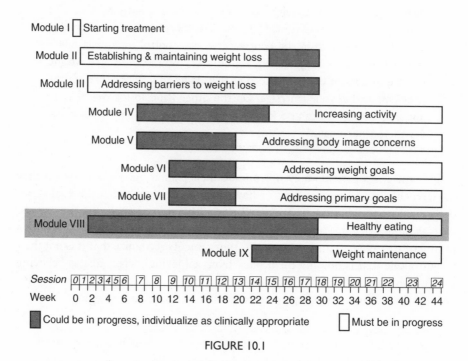

FIGURE 10.1

This module focuses on helping patients to eat healthily. It is relevant to all patients. It may be introduced at any time in treatment, but for patients who have a particularly high-fat diet, it should be introduced early on (see Figure 10.1). In our experience, many patients already know that in order to lose weight they should follow the guidelines described below, and while losing weight they should adhere to them. However, once they have lost weight, they tend gradually to return to their previous eating habits. With such patients this module can be delayed and entered at the same time as the module on long-term weight maintenance (see Chapter 11); indeed, it can be viewed as one aspect of weight maintenance. Even if these guidelines on healthy eating have been introduced earlier in treatment, therapists should return to them during the weight maintenance phase to ensure that patients understand the need to adhere to these principles in the long term.

This module focuses on two main topics, eating behavior and food choice.

1. *Eating behavior* (temporal pattern of eating, picking, portion sizes, etc.). All these topics will have already been covered earlier on in treatment (see Chapters 4 and 5). Nevertheless, the therapist should review each to see whether there are any residual problems to be addressed. If there are, they should be tackled using the same strategies as before.
2. *Food choice.* Up to this point in the treatment, food choice has only been addressed in the context of weight loss. The adoption of a healthy diet is an essential part of weight maintenance and as such it should become a focus of treatment at this point. A low-fat diet is recommended because it is a diet likely to facilitate successful long-term weight control, and it is the type of diet advocated for good overall health (in particular, the reduction in the risk of diseases such as coronary heart disease and various forms of cancer).

General Strategy for Encouraging Healthy Eating

To follow a low-fat diet the three key changes that most people are likely to have to make are as follows: reduce fat consumption; increase consumption of foods such as bread, cereal, rice, and pasta; and increase consumption of fruits and vegetables. The therapist needs to convey this information to patients and encourage them to follow these guidelines. In order to lose weight, many patients will have made some changes in line with these guidelines, but others may have continued to eat a relatively unhealthy diet and simply chosen to eat smaller quantities. Consequently the information provided must be tailored to the individual.

The overall strategy used to help patients make these changes is as follows:

1. *Explain the reasons for the recommendation.* The therapist should ensure that patients are clear about the reasons for each of the three dietary recommendations. Briefly they are as follows:

a. Reduce fat consumption:
- A low-fat diet is recommended for long-term weight maintenance. People who lose weight are less likely to regain the weight lost if they eat a low-fat diet, and those who eat low-fat diets tend to weigh less than those who do not.
- Fat contains twice as many calories per gram as protein or carbohydrates (i.e., it is "energy-dense"). It is therefore possible to eat a greater quantity of low-fat food for the same number of calories.
- A low-fat diet lowers blood cholesterol levels and so helps to reduce the risk of coronary disease.

b. Increase the consumption of bread, cereal, rice, and pasta:
- These foods provide energy and fiber. They are filling but low in fat.

- Consuming more of these foods ensures that calories from fat are decreased.

c. Increase the consumption of fruit and vegetables:

- These foods are high in fiber. They are filling but low in fat and so also ensure a decrease in calories from fat.
- Consuming more fruit and vegetables helps to lower the risk of developing heart disease.

2. *Assess current intake.* Once the patient understands the reasons for these dietary recommendations, it is necessary to assess the patient's diet to decide whether changes need to be made. This can be done by focusing on the last 3 days from the patient's food diaries and assessing each of the three areas in turn. As a guide to the therapist in conducting this assessment, current nutritional recommendations are as follows:

- No more than 35% of energy should be derived from fat.
- At least 11 portions of foods from the bread, cereal, rice, and pasta group should be consumed per day.
- Five portions of fruit and vegetables should be eaten.

We do not recommend asking patients to calculate precisely the amount of fat they are eating or the number of portions of particular foods they are eating. Instead, we suggest reviewing the patient's food diaries in general terms and discussing, if appropriate, the frequency with which the patient consumes foods that are high in fat, and the quantities eaten on each occasion. Similarly the discussions concerning bread, cereal, rice, and pasta, and fruit and vegetables should be conducted in the same general way, focusing on the amount of these foods eaten. In our view it is not helpful or practicable to ask patients to count exact portions of the various foods and doing so is likely to overburden them and put them at greater risk of abandoning their weight control efforts.

3. *Identify and agree areas for change.* Once the assessment of the patient's current intake has been completed, the patient and therapist need to agree which, if any, dietary changes are required and which the patient is prepared to try. The changes advocated should be realistic and achievable, they should fit in with food preferences, cooking ability, family likes and dislikes, budget, and so on, and be sustainable in the long term.

4. *Agree and plan clearly specified changes.* The patient and therapist should agree on specific achievable goals such as reducing portion size when eating meat, changing to a low-fat yogurt, or reducing fat intake by eating fewer fast-food meals. It may also be necessary to plan how these goals will be achieved—for example, to have quick and easy low-fat foods readily available so as to avoid eating fast food when busy.

A patient reviewed her diet with her therapist near the end of treatment. They considered the importance of a low-fat diet as part of a long-term strategy for weight maintenance. The patient described how, at the beginning of treatment, she had been diligent about ensuring everything she bought was as low as possible in fat, but, on examining her current intake, it was clear that she had started to eat a number of higher fat foods. The patient decided that there were some aspects of her diet that she did not want to change—for example, she had learned how to incorporate a moderate amount of chocolate into her diet without feeling she was breaking a dietary rule. However, there were other high-fat foods that she could easily reduce or eliminate altogether. She felt, for example, that to switch to lower-fat cheese would not affect her enjoyment of her food. She also resumed her previous practice of checking food labels, so that she could choose the lowest fat version of products. In addition, this patient also realized that a significant proportion of her fat intake came from fast food. Recently she had started to eat more of this. She agreed that some simple advance planning would solve this problem. She decided to eat fast food no more than once per week, and to plan meals in advance so she had quick and easy foods available for those days when she was busy.

---

5. *Review progress and address any difficulties.* Progress toward meeting agreed goals should always be reviewed and any problems addressed using the problem-solving approach described in Chapter 4.

6. *Long-term adherence to healthy eating.* Finally, the therapist needs to emphasize the importance of adhering to the principles of healthy eating in the long term. As noted earlier patients should be encouraged to make realistic changes that are sustainable in the long term. Patients should also be encouraged to devise an individualized plan for ensuring that they adhere to the changes they have made.

Having discussed the importance of eating a diet rich in bread, cereal, pasta, and rice, as well as increasing her consumption of fruit and vegetables, a patient was able to identify specific changes that would help her to achieve her goal of increasing her intake of these foods. In the past she had thought that the best way to keep her calorie intake under control was to have very small portions of rice, pasta, or potatoes, although she would eat whatever meat dishes were available regardless of their fat content. Following a discussion with her therapist, she attended a dinner party where she ate a moderate helping of rice, a side plate full of salad, both of which were foods she liked, and a small portion of the meat dish. She found this to be more satisfying, yet lower in calories and fat. Also she was pleased not to have to give up eating some of the meat dish because she wanted to be able to try it, and she did not want to stand out as being too fussy in her eating. She felt that this sort of change was one she could stick to in the long term, and after some practice she was able to regularly eat in this way both at home and on social occasions.

When reviewing another patient's fruit and vegetable intake, it was apparent that although she enjoyed these foods when she ate them, her daily intake was fairly low. As she liked these foods, she felt that she simply needed to make a more conscious effort to eat them each day. She decided that one change she could make would be to eat some exotic fruit as a snack instead of the chocolate she ate most days. By making sure that the fruit was readily available and appealing, she found it was a good substitute most of the time, and she ate chocolate as a snack more rarely. She also tried to make sure that she included some kind of fruit or vegetable at every meal. At breakfast she decided to have fruit juice or dried fruit with her cereal; she planned to take a salad to work to eat with her lunchtime sandwich; and even if she was having a quick evening meal, such as a prepared dish from the freezer, she decided she would boil some frozen vegetables to go with it or have a piece of fruit to follow. With these changes she found that her meals were much more satisfying and that she was much less likely to snack on other higher fat food.

CHAPTER 11

Module IX: Weight Maintenance

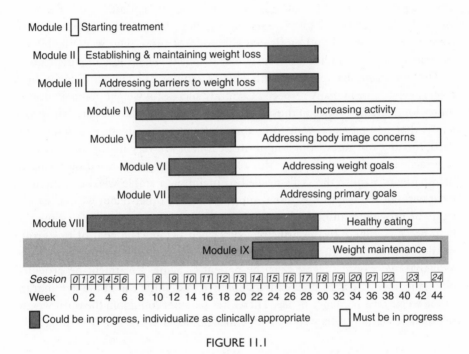

FIGURE 11.1

The most distinctive feature of this treatment is the priority it gives to weight maintenance. The subject is raised as an issue from the outset, and potential barriers to weight maintenance are identified and addressed at many different points as weight is lost—for example, when addressing unrealistic weight goals, primary goals, and body image dissatisfaction. Later in treatment, long-term weight maintenance becomes the primary focus.

The goals of this module are to help the patient to:

1. Prepare for weight maintenance.
2. Acquire the skills needed to maintain a stable weight in the long term.
3. Review progress in treatment.
4. Phase out self-monitoring.
5. Address the issue of weight change in the future.
6. Address how best to manage possible future attempts to lose weight.
7. Prepare a personal weight maintenance plan.

157

Obesity and Long-Term Care

Some authorities on obesity have recently argued that obesity should be viewed as a chronic disorder and that patients require long-term care (Perri & Corsica, 2002). There is some evidence that weight regain is delayed by longer treatment but not sufficient evidence about what happens when treatment eventually finishes. One of the few reports of successful weight maintenance with long-term support comes from a study of group support (Latner et al., 2000). A good long-term outcome was reported for those who continued to attend the support group. However, only 32% of those who began treatment attended for 3 years and only 22% attended for 5 years. In addition, those who began treatment were a highly selected and motivated subgroup of those who were eligible for treatment (60%), who had previously met stringent weight loss requirements.

The argument that patients with obesity require ongoing care in the long term is persuasive in many respects. Certainly successful weight maintenance requires long-term vigilance in those individuals predisposed to obesity. The problem is that few patients want to continue attending treatment indefinitely. Indeed, the dropout rates from long-term treatment are very high and increase as treatment is prolonged. It is for this reason that we have focused on trying to help patients acquire the skills needed to maintain a stable weight in the long term without the need for external support. On the other hand, we can see the value of providing an open, long-term weight maintenance group designed to help patients adhere to the principles described below. The goal of this group would be weight maintenance, not weight loss. Even if such a group were to be available, we would suggest that the patient's "acute" treatment be provided along the lines described here with it coming to a definite end at the termination of the weight maintenance phase. Thereafter patients could join the open weight maintenance group if they so wished, either immediately or at a later stage.

Determining When to Enter the Weight Maintenance Module

The weight maintenance module should be entered well before the end of treatment (see Figure 11.1). Our practice has been to allow at least 14 weeks for this phase of treatment. This is in order to allow sufficient time for patients to practice and consolidate their weight maintenance skills. It is preferable to enter the module even earlier than this (in our practice any time after week 20) to allow even longer to establish these skills. This is certainly indicated under either one of the following two circumstances:

1. If patients reach a point at which they do not wish to lose any more weight
2. If their weight loss has slowed down or ceased and, on discussion, the "costs" of attempting to lose further weight appear to outweigh the possible benefits

Once the weight maintenance module has been entered, weight maintenance remains the primary focus of the remainder of the treatment.

Overview of the Module

Patients need to be prepared for the process of weight maintenance, and this preparation should take place well in advance of the time at which they will be asked to stop trying to lose weight. This preparatory work is described in the section "Preparing for Weight Maintenance." On entering the weight maintenance phase, the sections "Defining a Target Weight Range and Establishing a Weight Monitoring System" and "Interpreting Changes in Weight" should be addressed immediately in the first two sessions. A considerable amount of time is then devoted in subsequent sessions to the sections "Developing Long-Term Weight Maintenance Skills" and "Responding to Changes in Weight." These sections cover the principles and practice of weight maintenance.

At some point during the module, therapists should help patients review their progress since starting treatment. The aim is both to identify what has been achieved and to assess what remains to be done. These topics are discussed in the section "Reviewing Treatment." Toward the end of treatment, the self-monitoring of food intake needs to be phased out ("Phasing Out Self-Monitoring"). The therapist should provide guidance about the topics "Addressing Weight Change in the Future" and "Possible Future Attempts to Lose Weight." Finally a personal weight maintenance plan should be devised and given to the patient ("Preparing a Personal Weight Maintenance Plan") together with a supply of weight maintenance graphs.

Throughout the weight maintenance phase of treatment, the sessions should retain the same structure as before with initial weighing, a review of progress, the setting of an agenda, and then working through the agenda. The main emphasis is on weight maintenance although primary goals will often continue to be addressed (see Chapter 9), and other modules may also be running in parallel (see Figure 11.1).

The final few sessions should become progressively more future oriented with therapists helping patients focus on how they will deal with future problems. Difficulties that have cropped up between sessions also need to be addressed from this perspective, with patients being encouraged to consider how they would tackle similar problems following the end of treatment.

Preparing for Weight Maintenance

Prior to embarking upon weight maintenance, therapists should have one or more preparatory discussions about the need to focus on weight maintenance. The following points need to be covered:

- There are many different ways to lose weight, but none to date has succeeded in helping people maintain their new, lower weight in the long term. Indeed, most treatments barely address weight maintenance, and if they do, it is sometimes more as an afterthought than as a focus of treatment in its own right. This treatment aims to help people develop, practice, and firmly establish the skills needed to maintain a stable weight.
- Most people who lose weight find that after 6 months of attempting to lose weight, their weight loss slows down and then stops (Wadden et al., 1999; Wilson & Brownell, 2002). Therefore, we encourage people to stop trying to lose weight at this point, and instead to concentrate their efforts on learning how to minimize the risk of regaining the weight that they have lost.
- To develop, practice, and establish weight maintenance skills, a significant period of time needs to be devoted to the issue. *It is essential that attempts to lose further weight are abandoned while doing this because they are not compatible with learning to maintain a new stable weight.*
- In our view, it is advisable that a period of learning weight maintenance skills be followed by a minimum of 6 months further practice at maintaining a stable weight.

Some patients will enter the weight maintenance phase reluctantly because they still weigh more than they would like to (i.e., "acceptance" remains a problem; see Chapter 8). Such patients need special help to cease their attempts to lose further weight. For them, the importance of learning to keep their weight stable must be stressed. The option of attempting to lose further weight in 9 months (i.e., after 3 months of supervised weight maintenance training followed by 6 months of self-directed practice) may be mentioned. Despite this, there are occasional patients who are unwilling to delay their weight loss attempts for as long as 9 months. The therapist should encourage such patients to think through the advantages and disadvantages of delaying their weight loss attempts. Patients should be encouraged to list these and discuss them in detail with the therapist. The therapist should help the patient evaluate these advantages and disadvantages in an objective and even-handed way, taking both a short-term perspective and a longer term one.

These preparatory points need to be restated in the first weight maintenance session. In addition, the steps involved in "training" in weight maintenance should be outlined. These are as follows:

1. Defining the weight range to be maintained
2. Establishing a practicable weight monitoring system for use in the long term
3. Learning how to interpret weight changes
4. Maintaining a stable weight
5. Learning how to deal with setbacks

There should always be a discussion of the difficulties inherent in long-term weight maintenance and the difference between weight loss and weight maintenance. It is particularly important to acknowledge that weight maintenance is less reinforcing than weight loss, for four reasons:

1. The goal is *no* weight change rather than weight loss.
2. There may have to be acceptance of a weight (and shape) that were previously viewed as undesirable.
3. The process is for an indefinite period of time rather than being time limited.
4. Patients may receive little encouragement from others.

The therapist's goal is to help patients recognize that weight maintenance is the natural next step in treatment rather than something that is being forced upon them. The hope is that active weight maintenance becomes second nature rather than an effort.

A negative response to the prospect of weight maintenance is not uncommon. This may arise from lack of acceptance of weight (and, more importantly, shape); resentment over the need to develop weight maintenance skills; and being disheartened at the prospect of doing this forever. These negative reactions may be expressed as poor attendance at sessions or even dropping out, hostility directed at the therapist or treatment, or the abandonment of dietary restraint. Therapists should be on the alert for such reactions. They should provide patients with the opportunity to ventilate their feelings about weight maintenance, both in advance of entering this module and at various stages while working through the module.

Some patients are also concerned about the prospect of ending treatment. They may be worried about their ability to cope in the absence of ongoing support, and they may feel that they need someone to report back to if they are going to remain motivated. In such cases our strategy has been to discuss these concerns rather than ignore them. It is best if they are identified early on so that there is sufficient time to address them. If the topic has not come up already, the therapist should actively raise the issue of termination at a minimum of four sessions before treatment is due to end and should ask how the patient feels about this, allowing ample time for discussion. At every subsequent session the therapist should remind the patient how many sessions are left, and address any ongoing issues related to the ending of treatment. In addition, the therapist should take pains to help patients see what they have already achieved during treatment, and these achievements should be attributed to the patient's own efforts. All evidence of their competence should be stressed.

The therapist asked a patient how she was feeling about ending treatment. The patient explained that she was worried about the prospect and was concerned about her ability to cope independently. She had struggled at times in treatment, particularly because she had many problems in her family and she was worried that these would prevent her from being able to manage her weight successfully. The therapist responded by helping the patient identify everything that she had achieved, focusing particularly on the skills that the patient had developed and how she could use them in the future. The therapist and patient worked together on drawing up her maintenance plan so that she had a concrete guide to the strategies she could use in future difficult situations. They also discussed how else she could get support. Although the patient and therapist had not focused on treating the family problems, the patient had been able to express her feelings in sessions and had found this helpful. They therefore discussed alternative forms of support ranging from friends to formal counseling or therapy. The patient remained somewhat anxious about ending treatment but was able to appreciate that she had the skills needed to manage her weight and a maintenance plan to help her deal with difficult times. She also knew how to obtain help to deal with other problems in her life.

Toward the end of treatment another patient was asked how she felt about ending treatment. She explained that she felt anxious about it, fearing that she would slip back to her old habits and regain weight. The therapist asked her to describe as clearly as possible her prediction as to what would happen. In what situations did she think things might become difficult? How did she see herself responding? What would the consequences of this be for her?

The therapist and patient were then able to examine these scenarios in detail and consider possible coping strategies for each of them. They discussed practical ways of dealing with difficult situations, and also examined the patient's interpretation of such events. The patient and therapist rehearsed appropriate responses to a range of possible situations, including the patient's vision of the "worst case scenario" so that she eventually felt she had coping strategies in place to deal with any difficulties that might arise.

Defining a Target Weight Range and Establishing a Weight Monitoring System

The first point to stress with patients is that they should maintain their weight within a weight range rather than trying to keep to a specific weight. This is to allow for natural day-to-day and week-to-week fluctuations. Our experience suggests that this weight range should be 8 lb (4 kg) in magnitude, and in most cases the center of this range should be the patient's average weight over the

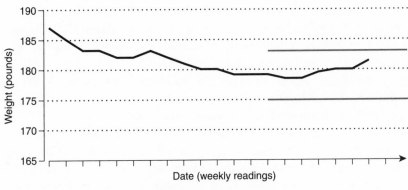

FIGURE 11.2 Example graph A

3 weeks prior to embarking on weight maintenance. This guideline needs to be modified in certain cases. For example some patients intensify their weight loss efforts in the weeks prior to weight maintenance with the goal of reaching as low a weight as possible. This can result in the choice of an inappropriately low weight range; that is, one that requires too much effort to maintain. The best way of dealing with this problem is to forestall it by discussing it in advance, but it might nevertheless be necessary to choose a slightly higher weight range.

Therapists must always give careful thought to the choice of weight range, and patients should be actively involved in the decision. Once the range has been selected, the therapist should highlight the upper and lower weight limits (which we refer to as "tramlines") in the appropriate place on the weight graph, and extend these lines to the end of treatment. Patients should be provided with a new maintenance graph for their use with their weight marked on it, and they should be asked to draw the tramlines on this graph (see Figure 11.2).

For successful weight maintenance, the patient needs to establish an appropriate weight monitoring system.[1] This should be capable of detecting significant weight changes, but it must also be practicable as it will have to be used indefinitely. In practice the following arrangement seems to work. Patients should weigh themselves once a week on a morning of their choice. (They are advised to choose a day that is likely to be most convenient or that they are most likely to remember—for example, Monday morning if they associate weighing themselves with part of their "starting the working week" routine). This routine weigh-in provides their "official" weight for the week. The patient should record the date and his or her weight on a long-term weight maintenance graph, which should be kept somewhere private but prominent—for example, on the

---

[1]By this stage in treatment, any difficulties patients may have had with weighing themselves will have been addressed (see Chapters 3 and 7). These include the active avoidance of weighing, too frequent weighing, and inappropriate rituals surrounding weighing.

inside of a closet door. (Until the end of treatment, the graph should be portable as patients will need to bring it to each appointment.) Patients should refer to their graph each week to look for signs of significant weight change in order to decide whether any action is indicated (see below).

In explaining the principles of weight monitoring, it is essential that therapists make it absolutely clear that patients will need to monitor their weight indefinitely. This is because of the continuing risk of weight regain.

Once the tramlines have been drawn, it should be explained that the patient's aim should be to keep his or her weight within them. This involves deciding not to attempt to lose any further weight. Indeed, from this stage on, weight loss is as undesirable (from the perspective of treatment) as weight gain, as it does not allow patients to learn how to keep their weight steady.

Many patients are anxious about identifying the appropriate calorie intake for weight maintenance. Interestingly, this is not as problematic as it sounds. Among the many patients whose weight loss has already ceased, there need be no change in energy intake (however low it *appears* to be from their records). Among patients who are continuing to lose weight, a slight relaxation of their dietary restriction should be recommended. Some patients request more specific guidance. Unfortunately, it is impossible to specify someone's exact energy requirements for day-to-day life, and because patients' recording is rarely absolutely accurate by this stage in treatment, doing so is unlikely to be useful anyway. Quoting population averages is rarely helpful due to inaccurate recording and individual differences. Sometimes guidance can be drawn from the patient's own experience. Records of weight during treatment can be reviewed to see if there was a time when the patient maintained rather than lost weight (such as during a vacation). Old food diaries can then be consulted to ascertain calorie intake at that time. All patients should be advised not to reduce their level of physical activity.

If a change in energy intake appears to be indicated, the therapist should guide the patient to make small changes (e.g., raising calorie goal by 100 calories per day if they have continued to lose weight slowly) and to monitor the effects on their weight, thus taking an experimental approach. For instance, a patient who had successfully lost weight on an apparent intake of 1,500 calories per day might be encouraged to aim for around 1,600 calories per day, and assess any change in weight over 2–3 weeks. At a minimum, a period of at least 2 weeks should elapse before any further changes are made.

The need to relax dietary controls—but not abandon them—merits careful discussion. This is to counter the widely held belief that once one has finished losing weight, one can return to one's old eating habits. The therapist needs to explain that, to maintain their current weight, patients will have to eat less than they did prior to treatment. This is in part because they may have been gaining weight before starting treatment (i.e., they were in positive energy balance), and in part because they are now lighter than they were and so daily energy requirements are lower. In practice it is not uncommon for patients to increase their food intake and gain a little weight. The chances of this happening can be reduced by warning them in advance that their weight is likely to rise a little if they increase their calorie intake by more than a very small amount (e.g., the equivalent of one extra banana a day). Sometimes there is a period of trial and error while patients adjust their food intake to stabilize their weight.

Homework at the end of this first session of weight maintenance should be to:

1. monitor weight in the way described;
2. bring their weight graph to the next session;
3. stop attempting to lose further weight, and, if necessary, adjust calorie intake to maintain a stable weight.

After the first 2 weeks in weight maintenance, a patient had shown a small increase in weight and her calorie intake was higher than the provisional goal that she had set for herself. When guiding the therapist through her diaries she explained that she had experienced a temporary abandoning of control in the excitement of having been "freed" from the restriction imposed by the goal of weight loss. However, she had quickly recognized that weight maintenance could not be equated with the abandonment of control—it simply offered a degree of flexibility beyond that which had been possible while she was losing weight. She subsequently moderated her eating to establish a pattern that was consistent with weight maintenance.

Another patient commented after her first 2 weeks of weight maintenance (at which she had been very successful), that she was disappointed by the low calorie level that seemed to be required for her to maintain her weight. She had recorded an average daily intake of 1,600 calories over the 2-week period, and prior to that had been losing weight on 1,500 calories per day. The patient explained that she had enjoyed her food over the last 2 weeks and had noticed the extra flexibility afforded by the slight increase in calories. She had been able to eat more fruit and had found it easier to manage her intake when eating socially. However, she commented, "If I can only eat 1,600 calories a day for the rest of my life that is depressing, because I still feel restricted. I can balance out my calories to allow for higher days by cutting back on other days, I suppose, but it just does not seem to add up. I lost weight on 1,500 calories, and increasing by just 100 calories a day I am now maintaining my weight. Why should it be such a small increase?"

The therapist responded with several points. First, although the patient felt dissatisfied with the number of calories she was consuming, she seemed to be enjoying the food itself. In other words it appeared that it was not the actual quantity of food on the plate that troubled her, but the thought that it was not enough. The therapist also commented that, because the patient had eaten out several times over the last 2 weeks, her calorie totals on those days were presumably "best guesses," thereby making the numbers less reliable. The therapist also noted that, despite doing her best to be accurate with her calorie counting, the patient needed to remember that most people underestimate their calorie intake, and she might well be eating more than 1,600 calories per day. The therapist suggested that the patient might feel happier if she focused on the fact that she had eaten well and enjoyed herself when eating out, rather than worry about the exact number of calories she was "allowed."

There were several other issues that the therapist thought were worth discussing in this context:

- It was too early in weight maintenance to be sure if this was an appropriate long-term calorie goal. Further experience would be needed.
- An increase in physical activity (if not already achieved) can allow a slight increase in calorie intake and might therefore be a goal worth aiming for during maintenance. On the other hand, this could not be relied on as a core strategy because the additional energy expenditure from physical activity is modest.
- Choosing low-fat foods greatly increases the quantity of food that can be eaten without increasing the calorie content. The therapist recommended several good low-fat cookbooks.
- The patient would need to come to terms with the fact that her energy maintenance requirements would never be as high as they were prior to her weight loss. She could never expect to return to her previous way of eating, if she was going to avoid weight regain.
- Even "normal"-weight people have to be aware of, and to some extent control, their food intake. Some degree of "restriction" is therefore inevitable.

At the next session, the therapist suggested that this might be a suitable time for the patient to start phasing out her monitoring of food intake (see below). The patient therefore kept food records for the next 2 weeks but discontinued counting calories. She continued to be successful at maintaining her weight within the tramlines, and from the following session onward she ceased recording her food intake altogether. During this process the patient came to learn that thinking about the number of calories that she ate was not helpful to her. Rather, focusing on the food that she was eating, and the level of flexibility she now had (as compared to when she was losing weight), helped her to feel satisfied with what she was eating.

Interpreting Changes in Weight

Patients need to learn to distinguish significant changes in their weight from trivial weight fluctuations. With this in mind, patients should be taught to be on the alert for any one of following three phenomena:

1. *Their weight moving outside the tramlines.* If this occurs the patient must take stock (see below).

2. *A weight trend suggestive of weight regain.* Here the challenge is distinguishing such a trend from background fluctuations in weight. Week-to-week fluctuations within the tramlines are of little note; although, if their amplitude increases, this is suggestive of instability in the patient's eating (which might put him or her at risk of weight regain). To identify a trend suggestive of weight regain, the patient should focus not only on how weight has changed since the last recording, but also on changes over the past 4 weeks. Patients should therefore be advised to concentrate on their last four readings and examine whether they reveal evidence of weight regain.[2] Sample weight graphs are shown in Figures 11.2, 11.3, and 11.4.

Figure 11.2 shows a trend toward weight regain, which should be addressed; Figure 11.3 illustrates successful weight maintenance (no trend upward or downward over the past four readings); whereas Figure 11.4 illustrates ongoing weight loss, which should be addressed, as it will prevent the patient from learning how to maintain a stable weight.

3. *A sudden change in weight.* Sudden changes in weight also need to be thought about and, if necessary, acted upon. For example, weight loss following an acute illness needs to be monitored although it may not require action. In contrast, sudden gain in weight due to the resumption of binge eating re-

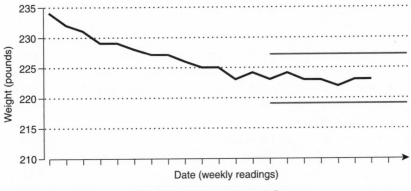

FIGURE 11.3 Example graph B

---

[2]Some female patients experience significant premenstrual weight gain. If this pattern is clear and consistent, it should be taken into account when interpreting weight fluctuations. This will require discussion with the therapist and practice during this final phase of treatment.

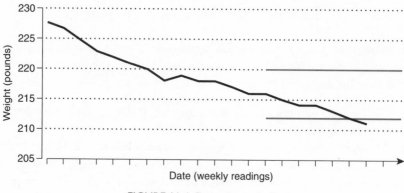

FIGURE 11.4 Example graph C

quires urgent attention. Any weight change (over two consecutive readings) of 4.5 lb (2.0 kg) or greater is of concern.

At the beginning of each weight maintenance session, therapists should ask patients to comment on the significance of the latest reading. This involves plotting their weight on their personal weight graph (while the therapist does the equivalent), and looking for any of the three phenomena noted above. In this way the therapist helps the patient develop skills in recognizing significant changes. The patient also needs to do the same following each between-session weighing.

Developing Long-Term Weight Maintenance Skills

Therapists should devote a considerable amount of time to discussion of the principles of long-term weight maintenance. These are as follows:

- *Successful weight maintenance requires balancing energy intake with energy expenditure.* Controlling energy intake is the more important of the two as it has greater influence on weight regain; although physical activity must not be neglected because clinical experience and research evidence suggest that those people who maintain an active lifestyle are best at weight maintenance.
- *Patients need to practice maintaining their weight over a range of circumstances* including vacations, times of stress, and periods of ill health or enforced inactivity. Some of these circumstances may be predictable (e.g., vacations) and are therefore amenable to advance planning. Others are unpredictable and may only be open to corrective action after the event.
- *Weight needs to be regularly monitored and evaluated* in the manner already described. This will need to be done indefinitely.
- *Changes in weight are almost always due to a change in energy intake or activity level, or both.* Exceptions are pregnancy and the influence of cer-

tain illnesses (e.g., thyroid disease, diabetes mellitus, cancer) and drugs (e.g., steroids, some antidepressant and antipsychotic drugs).

- *Correcting for changes in weight involves either a change in energy intake or a change in expenditure, or both.* Changing energy intake is the more potent of the two methods.

- *There is evidence that those people who maintain an active lifestyle are most successful at weight maintenance.* Although the nature of the relationship between the two has not been established, this finding is sufficient to justify encouraging patients to adopt an active lifestyle.

- *Significant weight change must be spotted and promptly addressed.* See discussion below of the relative merits of maintaining a stable weight in the center of the target range, as opposed to allowing small weight gains, which are corrected when necessary.

- *Once weight has returned to the target range, there needs to be a further correction of energy intake or expenditure (or both) to maintain the new weight.* This further reinforces the need for careful ongoing monitoring of weight.

In addition, all patients should be asked to consider the following questions:

- *What are the relative merits of making an effort to maintain a weight around the center of the tramlines, compared with allowing weight to go up until it reaches the upper tramline, and then making the necessary corrections?* Patients should be encouraged to list the advantages and disadvantages of these two different strategies. Some patients think that they would prefer to be more relaxed and eat whatever they want until their weight reaches the top tramline; at which point they would start to record their calorie intake again and reduce their food intake until their weight has returned to the center of the tramlines. However, after consideration, most patients acknowledge that such a strategy would be difficult, as it would involve repeatedly going on a restrictive diet, which could be discouraging. Also, many will know from past experience that weight gain of this kind can be so disheartening that it is likely to put them at greater risk of abandoning their weight control effort altogether. This is particularly likely to be a risk if patients still tend to think in dichotomous ("black-and-white") terms. It is generally easier to get used to eating roughly the same amount, so that the choices become second nature, rather than swaying from one eating pattern to another. It may be useful to refer to the patient's past experience of strategies that have been useful and those that have not.

- *Is it worth thinking ahead?* Patients should be encouraged to be on the alert for times when there is increased risk of weight gain (e.g., vacations and festivities). They should be asked to consider the relative merits of avoiding weight gain at these times (but still having a good time) as against letting weight gain occur and then having to compensate for it.

- *Are there aspects of the patient's behavior or attitudes that put him or her at particular risk of weight regain?* These might include a proclivity to eat high-fat snacks when under stress, a tendency to be less active during the winter, the view that when on vacation one should be able to eat whatever one likes, a tendency to overeat when eating out, and so on. Patients should be asked to think through the implications of these vulnerabilities for successful weight maintenance in the long term. Are there any changes that the patient should consider? Is there anything that they might usefully practice?

One patient lost 13% of her initial body weight in the first 6 months of treatment. At this point, the issue of weight maintenance arose. Although the patient had been aware of the weight maintenance phase from the outset of treatment, she became upset at the idea of having to stop losing weight. From this point on, her weight loss began to slow down, and the patient appeared despondent about the prospect of eventually finishing treatment. She felt that she had not lost enough weight and that she had not "changed enough." She continued to have a poor body image, despite attempts to address this issue in treatment.

The patient reluctantly agreed to commence weight maintenance. She maintained her weight for 2 weeks, but, over the next few weeks, she gradually regained weight. She was advised to take immediate action, including recommencing self-monitoring (which she had started to phase out) and limiting her calorie intake to 1,500 calories again. She struggled to achieve these goals.

There appeared to be several reasons for her difficulties with weight maintenance. First, she remained very unhappy with her current weight and appearance, and she was resistant to the idea of weight maintenance as opposed to further weight loss. Second, she continued to think of herself as either "on" or "off" a diet, and she had little experience of following a regular, healthy eating pattern. Related to this was her reluctance to modify her food choice: she had retained a strong preference for high-calorie foods. Third, she had also found it difficult to address her primary goals—she was reluctant to try to increase her social contacts until she had lost more weight because she felt that people would make fun of her. She had become "stuck" in a vicious circle.

Another patient found that social eating was making it difficult for her to stick to her calorie goal. She often entertained friends at home, or ate at their houses or in restaurants. She was loath to discuss her dietary requirements with her friends, as she preferred to keep her weight control efforts private. The therapist questioned her about how she would feel if a friend asked her to provide a meal to suit his or her dietary needs. She replied that she would be eager to accommodate such wishes and would even be upset if the friend did not ask her. However, she still did not feel that asking others to plan their menus around her needs was a strategy that she could employ. She discussed alternative possibilities with her therapist; for instance, taking small portions, refusing second helpings, and making careful choices in restaurants. She initially appeared reluctant to employ these strategies. It seemed that social eating was such an important aspect of her life that change was difficult. The therapist continued to encourage her to try these techniques and praised her for any attempts she made to stick to her calorie goal when eating socially. As time went by, the patient became better at coping with social eating. The first major breakthrough was her discovery that she could cook delicious dinner party dishes that were low in calories, so that at least when she was entertaining she could make sure there was always a suitable choice. She also became adept at serving cream and sauces separately so she could avoid them if she chose. She began to find it easier to ask for smaller portions and refuse second helpings when she ate with friends. She also learned which dishes on restaurant menus were good choices for her, and she took to "banking calories" on either side of special meals to give herself greater flexibility.

• *What is the patient's likely reaction to a change in weight and is it likely to make matters worse?* For example, patients should consider whether they might be tempted to stop monitoring their weight (i.e., turn a blind eye); whether they might be prone to hope that the problem will go away of its own accord (i.e., wishful thinking); or might they give up their attempts at weight control altogether (i.e., black-and-white thinking)? Therapists should ask patients to consider all these possibilities and how they might usefully be addressed.

Responding to Changes in Weight

Next patients need to learn the steps involved in responding to significant changes in weight. These are summarized below and discussed in detail in the handout "Responding to Change in Weight" (Handout U), which the therapist should work through with the patient. Below are the main points to cover.

1. *Identifying and evaluating any change in weight:*
   • Is it a sudden leap or a gradual trend?
   • Is weight now outside the tramlines?

2. *Identifying the explanation for any change in weight (in terms of energy intake and expenditure).* Consider reasons for the change:
   • A change in eating
   • A change in activity
   • Ill health, pregnancy, or medication

Common causes of weight gain include an insidious increase in portion size (which often goes undetected), picking at food, a change in food choice (with increased intake of energy-dense foods), and stress-related eating. Changes in both lifestyle and more formal exercise should be considered as well.

3. *Identifying the background cause(s) of any change in behavior:*
   - Is there an obvious explanation for the change?
   - Is it due to a change in habits?

4. *Devising and implementing a plan for addressing the weight gain.* Patients should be encouraged to devise a plan for correcting the weight gain. There will need to be two phases: First, an energy deficit needs to be established to bring weight back into the middle of the tramlines. This will usually involve restricting food intake for some weeks (to, say, 1,500 calories). Progress needs to be carefully monitored (e.g., every 3 or 7 days) and strategy adjusted accordingly. Second, once the weight change has been corrected, further adjustments will be needed to stabilize weight. Generally these will involve changes in both energy intake and physical activity following the guidelines that have been provided. Monitoring of food intake will have to be discontinued, but regular monitoring of weight should continue.

5. *Devising and implementing a plan for dealing with the background cause(s) of the change in behavior.* Patients also need to address the background cause of the weight gain. This is best done using the formal problem-solving approach (see Chapter 4). As with the changes in eating and activity, progress should be regularly evaluated and plans adjusted accordingly.

One year after completing treatment, a patient's weight began to creep up. Initially, she found it difficult to identify the cause. Through detailed self-monitoring she identified that she was now eating bigger portions, picking at food in the evenings, and less active than she had been 6 months earlier. There seemed to be several reasons for this. One was that it was now winter, and she was staying in rather than gardening or going for walks in the evening. Another was that she had a new partner and he liked to snack while watching television. He also ate large meals, which might have contributed to the increase in the size of her portions.

Another patient who had struggled throughout treatment with a black-and-white thinking style presented at one weight maintenance session having gained 4 lb (1.8 kg). This took her close to the top of her tramlines. Until that point she had maintained her weight almost without fluctuation. She was distressed about her weight gain. Her weight had started to increase after a period of illness, which had coincided with low mood. In her first weekly review of this period, she identified that she felt helpless, hopeless, and ill, but she reminded herself that she needed to be assertive regarding her food and that it would be possible for her to eat moderately and still be "kind to herself." A few days later, she resumed recording her food intake following a "mini-review" in which she decided to carefully assess her calorie intake. She weighed herself, and, although her weight had increased again, she used the information constructively to motivate herself. She was aware that it was important for her not to feel devastated by what was, in reality, a minor lapse. She began to appreciate that learning to deal with weight changes was integral to weight maintenance, and as such it was a positive experience. She acknowledged that although premenstrual weight gain was in part responsible for the increase in her weight, she had also been overeating, and she needed to take appropriate action to combat this. Hence her decision to resume recording. Her second decision was to wait rather than panic or try to take dramatic corrective action. She also reminded herself that her weight gain did not indicate that she was a "bad person" or a "failure" in any way.

The therapist congratulated her on achieving all this and emphasized how important it was to see the present experience as a learning opportunity. The therapist also encouraged her to interpret weight fluctuations neutrally (i.e., as a result of a change in energy intake or expenditure and/or some other physiological change) rather than as evidence of personal failure. The patient was able to bring her weight back down toward the center of the tramlines, and she continued to become more accepting of minor fluctuations in her weight.

Reviewing Treatment

At some point during this final phase in treatment, it is good practice to help patients review their overall progress. There are two aims. The first is to identify what has been achieved, which often gets forgotten. The second aim is to assess what remains to be done, either during treatment or afterward. Sometimes it is helpful to look back at old monitoring records, questionnaires, and checklists. When there are outstanding issues (e.g., concerning activity or body image), the therapist should try to address these in treatment, if time allows. Otherwise, therapists should help patients construct plans for addressing them in the future.

Phasing Out Self-Monitoring

Toward the end of treatment, patients need to discontinue monitoring their eating. It is unrealistic to expect them to continue monitoring indefinitely. It is best if patients stop monitoring during treatment, rather than suddenly stopping at the very end of treatment (or at some other point in the future when it becomes too burdensome) when they are likely to be at increased risk of relapse. This helps patients to adjust to the change while still receiving support from the therapist. It is also valuable to have patients practice maintaining their weight while not monitoring their food intake.

We recommend that the discontinuation of monitoring be done in steps. Our practice is to introduce the first step at least six sessions before the end of treatment, with the second step following at the next session.

Step 1. Ask patients to stop recording their calorie intake but to continue writing down the food that they consume. Ask them to predict the likely consequences of doing this, and devise a plan for dealing with difficulties that are likely to arise as a result.

Step 2. Review the impact of this change on eating and weight. Unless there have been serious difficulties (e.g., a rapid weight increase), ask patients to stop monitoring their eating altogether. Ask them to predict the likely consequences of doing so and devise a plan for dealing with any difficulties that are likely to occur. (If there have been difficulties with step 1, these should be addressed using a problem-solving approach (see Chapter 4), with step 2 being delayed until the next session).

Step 3. Review the impact on eating and weight of stopping recording altogether.

Patients vary in their response to the prospect of phasing out recording. One patient had mixed feelings. She felt concerned that not recording would make it difficult for her to control her intake, but she was aware that it was not realistic to continue monitoring indefinitely. The therapist and patient discussed her concerns, and the pros and cons of discontinuing recording earlier rather than later in treatment. The patient felt that the best thing she could do was to take control, and test out how things would be without records. She decided to stop recording calories for 1 week, reassess the situation at her weekly review and, if she felt comfortable, to then stop recording altogether. She did this, and noted after the first week that she had not missed recording at all—she began to wonder how she had managed to keep it up for 9 months! She had envisaged her weight sky-rocketing as soon as she stopped recording but was pleased to find it remained stable. Although she felt that she had overeaten on occasions, she was able to conclude on the basis of evidence gathered over a few weeks that her weight had not gone up and that perhaps she had not overeaten significantly. Her confidence was boosted by this experience, and she progressed well in weight maintenance, using records only occasionally when she felt that she needed to regain control.

Another patient had ceased to record some weeks prior to the start of weight maintenance. The patient and therapist discussed the relative merits of resuming recording on a temporary basis in order to establish what might be a suitable calorie intake for weight maintenance. Although the patient could see this might be helpful, she was reluctant to resume recording, feeling that she had already learned to adjust her intake on the basis of quantity and type of food consumed rather than number of calories. The patient and therapist agreed that she would continue without recording on an experimental basis. If she found it difficult to maintain her weight, recording could be reinstated. The weight maintenance phase went well with the patient only monitoring on one occasion when she experienced a slight gain in weight.

A third patient was extremely distressed at the prospect of giving up recording. She became tearful when the issue was raised. She feared that giving up recording would result in her losing control completely. The therapist encouraged her to try it out as an experiment, on the basis that it would be better to try it sooner rather than later. In this way, if anything did go wrong, there would be plenty of time within treatment to sort things out. The patient initially tried to stop counting calories. In order to cope, she instituted a rigid "balancing system," such that if she felt the types of foods she had eaten were too high in fat or calories, she would compensate the next day by eating very little. At her next session, the therapist asked her about this balancing system, and the patient began to see that although "balancing" might be a good idea in principle, being rigid and extreme about it put her at risk of setting up a "see-saw" pattern of overeating and then undereating. In spite of her concerns, she had not lost control. The therapist then suggested that she stop recording altogether. The patient remained anxious. She explained that she would find it really difficult to manage her intake without making reference to the nutrition labels on foods, and taking some account of their calorie content. The therapist explained that the idea was not to abandon all interest in the energy content of foods, but simply to stop keeping detailed written records. The therapist reassured the patient that many people do keep an "eye on" their food consumption, as part of remaining conscious of their health. The patient felt reassured by this and agreed to stop recording. She found that she was able to keep track of her intake by means other than formal recording. Her weight remained stable in spite of her fears about losing control.

Addressing Weight Change in the Future

Toward the end of treatment, patients should be asked to consider how they would deal with certain specific difficulties in the future. They will already have learned in principle the steps involved in responding to changes in weight. The focus at this stage should be on helping patients plan exactly how they would react to any weight change. Relevant scenarios for discussion include the following:

• *The patient returns from a 2-week vacation to discover that his or her weight has increased by 4 lb (2 kg) and is now on the upper tramline.* In this situation there are two issues to discuss: first, whether it might have been preferable to ensure that this weight gain did not occur; and second, what should be done if the patient experiences this situation. The therapist should ask the patient to consider whether abandoning weight control while on vacation is a helpful strategy or not. The therapist should ensure that the patient considers the long-term effects of not being vigilant about weight while on vacation (i.e., that it may contribute to inadvertent weight gain that can take months to reverse and that it may result in the patient's feeling demoralized and giving up any weight control efforts altogether). The therapist should help the patient to consider alternative strategies such as planning ahead for vacations, following the guidelines in Handout H ("Planning for Vacations").

Should patients discover that their weight has risen to the upper tramline (or above it) while they have been on vacation (whether or not this was anticipated), they should be encouraged to deal with the weight gain following the principles already discussed. They should begin to record their food intake again and adhere to an appropriate calorie goal (e.g., 1,500 calories /day), until their weight has returned to the center of the tramlines.

• *The patient finds on routine weighing that his or her weight appears to be creeping up.* Patients should be encouraged to follow the strategies learned in treatment and summarized in Handout U ("Responding to Changes in Weight"). If weight has risen above the top tramline, they should be encouraged to resume recording their calorie intake and keep to an appropriate calorie goal. If their weight has been creeping up over the previous few weeks but is still within the tramlines, they should consider what might have changed (in their calorie intake or activity) to have caused this, and they should take appropriate action to reverse the trend.

• *The patient breaks a leg and is immobilized for some weeks. The broken leg is in a cast and as a result the patient cannot weigh himself or herself.* Patients should be encouraged to assess the risks that may be involved in this or a similar situation and how they would keep a check on their weight. Issues to consider include: They may be around food more than usual; they may feel bored or fed up, and so be prone to eat more; people might bring them chocolates or other treats; and their activity level is likely to be very low. A further point to consider is that when the cast is removed, the patient may be lighter than expected due to muscle wastage, but this weight will be regained as muscle is built up again. Patients should be encouraged to use their problem-solving skills to devise a plan for such eventualities. For example, in this instance would it be possible for them to weigh themselves while in the cast to get a new baseline weight, then weigh again each week to monitor any change?

• *The patient is ill or under stress (e.g., due to family illness, problems at work, financial difficulties) and the patient's weight falls below the lower tramline.* Patients should be helped to consider whether weight loss is helpful in this situation. A particularly important issue to consider is whether weight loss at this stage interferes with acquiring and practicing the skills to maintain a steady weight. Patients also need to consider the reasons for a drop in their weight, and whether an immediate reaction (in the form of overeating in an attempt to regain the lost weight) is required. After times of stress or illness, patients usually find that weight is regained without a deliberate effort. The therapist should help the patient to reach the conclusion that deliberately attempting to lose weight during this time is unhelpful.

A patient who was in the weight maintenance phase of treatment was ill for a time. Once she had recovered, she noted that her weight had dropped below the bottom tramline. She discussed the situation with her therapist, uncertain as to whether she should deliberately attempt to gain weight to get herself back to the center of the tramlines. As a result of this discussion, she decided to continue to eat at a maintenance level and monitor her weight rather than changing anything immediately. They discussed how a period of illness can result in rapid weight loss, but that this weight is often rapidly regained once the person starts eating and drinking normally. The patient did indeed notice a slight increase in weight, but, after another 2 weeks of eating according to her usual maintenance pattern, her weight had only just crept over the lower tramline. The patient and therapist reviewed the situation and agreed that if the patient's weight was stable and she was eating as she had been prior to her illness (at which time she had been maintaining her weight around the center of the tramlines), it would not be helpful to try to gain weight simply to get back to her previous position. Instead, they agreed that it would make sense for her to aim to continue to maintain her weight near the lower tramline.

• *The patient gives birth and is significantly heavier than she was before her pregnancy.* During pregnancy the patient should be encouraged to seek advice about healthy eating. She should be aware that the popular saying that a pregnant woman needs to "eat for two" is a myth, and the actual increase in energy consumption required during pregnancy is fairly small, and only applies to the later stages of pregnancy (see Rössner, 2002). After giving birth, the patient should be encouraged to review her situation with the aim of gradually trying to return to the eating habits she had established during the weight maintenance period of treatment. Patients should again be encouraged to use problem-solving skills to help them address any lifestyle changes that might interfere with this strategy (e.g., being at home with a baby instead of out of the house). Patients should be encouraged to consider what is a reasonable activity level for them and how this can be achieved on a sustainable basis, and how best to continue to monitor their weight. The widely held view that breastfeeding is associated with greater weight loss is not strictly accurate.

As homework the patient should be encouraged to think of other situations that they might experience that would put them at risk of gaining weight, and how they would cope with them. Other scenarios that might be discussed include giving up smoking[3]; retiring from work or having a career change; a family crisis; becoming unemployed; looking after young children at home; spending a period of time in the hospital; and, for women, going through menopause, and starting hormone replacement therapy. In each instance, strategies should be discussed and specific plans developed. Particularly relevant scenarios should be included in the weight maintenance plan (see below).

Addressing Possible Future Attempts to Lose Weight

Some patients will want to try to lose more weight in the future. This possibility needs to be addressed as trying to lose further weight may result in adverse consequences. If patients set themselves a weight goal that is unlikely to be achieved, there is a danger that they will feel they have failed if they do not achieve this goal. They are also at risk of undervaluing what they *have* achieved. As a result they may abandon any efforts to maintain their new weight, or, at least, they may only attempt to maintain it in a half-hearted fashion because they do not believe that they have controlled their weight to any worthwhile extent. Even if patients achieve a weight with which they are satisfied, if they need to exercise extreme dietary restraint in order to maintain this weight, there is a danger that they will not succeed in keeping this up in the

---

[3]Smoking, like obesity, is a major health risk. Sometimes patients decide that because they are making healthy lifestyle changes, they would also like to give up smoking. This is a positive step in terms of health and should be welcomed. With patients who ask whether they should stop smoking, we recommend that therapists inform them that:

- stopping smoking has definite health benefits and is a good idea;
- it may not be a good idea to attempt to stop smoking during the early stages of treatment (the first 6 weeks), as they are already attempting to make many major lifestyle changes, and it can be difficult to make so many changes at one time;
- ceasing smoking is generally associated with some weight gain, but if patients stick to the weight management techniques introduced during treatment, this is unlikely to happen;
- if they want further help, they should contact their physician or organizations that specialize in helping people stop smoking.

long term. Our clinical experience indicates that once some weight gain occurs and it becomes clear that it is not possible to maintain the desired low weight, many patients abandon all attempts at weight control (viewing it as too difficult and as not producing the desired benefits).

When addressing the desire to lose further weight, patients should be encouraged to consider why they want to lose weight and whether losing weight will help them achieve what they want. They may be confusing "primary goals" (e.g., to find more friends or a partner) with the desire to lose weight, and there may be something else they could more usefully do. They should consider whether the benefits of further weight loss are really greater than the considerable effort involved in losing the weight.

In discussing these issues, patients should be reminded to consider whether premature attempts to lose weight may interfere with the acquisition of weight maintenance skills. They should be advised that, in our experience, it is best to postpone further attempts to lose weight for at least 6 months following the end of treatment.

If patients are determined to try to lose more weight, the therapist should review with them how they intend to do this. If they have specific plans, these should be discussed with the aim of identifying any difficulties that might arise. Agreed strategies should be included in the weight maintenance plan (see below). In general, it is best to recommend the methods that have been used in treatment (i.e., recording calories consumed, using the same calorie goal they used in treatment, following the guidance on healthy eating, etc.).

Finally, patients should be reminded of the value of following any attempt to lose weight with a period of weight maintenance in order to "lock onto" their new weight. This point should be included in their personal weight maintenance plan (see below).

While discussing weight goals (see Chapter 8), a patient explained that her goal was to reach 133 lb (60.3 kg; BMI 22.4). At that stage in treatment (week 28), she had lost 24 lb (10.9 kg) and had reached a weight of 168 lb (76. 2 kg; BMI 28.3). She was happy to enter the maintenance phase of treatment but remained eager to progress toward her ultimate goal in the long term. The therapist was concerned that this was not a realistic goal as the patient's only previous experience of maintaining a weight as low as this had been at a time when she was eating very little, exercising heavily, and taking weight loss pills. Even then, she was unable to maintain this weight for long.

During the preparation of the patient's maintenance plan, the therapist raised this issue. In spite of the patient's prior experience of subsequent weight regain, she continued to express the firm intention to aim for this goal in the long term. As she was clearly not going to revise her goal, the therapist had to take a pragmatic approach. This involved educating the patient about the importance of only making further attempts at weight loss: (1) after consolidating her weight maintenance skills for at least 9 months; (2) for a time-defined period, then "locking on" to weight maintenance again; and (3) if, after due consideration, there was no other more appropriate way of achieving her personal goals. In this way the therapist hoped that the patient might work toward her ultimate goal, but in a stepwise fashion and without ever losing her weight maintenance skills. The patient and therapist included these notes in the maintenance plan and, by the end of treatment, the patient stated that she did intend to lose more weight eventually, but that she could appreciate the importance of consolidating her weight maintenance skills. She planned to review her options in approximately 6 months' time.

Preparing a Personal Weight Maintenance Plan

Toward the end of treatment, the therapist and patient should together draw up a personal weight maintenance plan. This generally takes three sessions, and so should be introduced by three sessions before the end at the latest. Each of the following steps can be covered in one session (with homework to be completed before the next one).

Step 1

First, the therapist should discuss the value of having an explicit and written plan, which provides detailed guidance about weight control in the future (the "weight maintenance plan"). The two main points to stress are that this plan can act as a useful reminder of what has been learned about weight maintenance, and it will provide detailed, personally relevant guidance about what to do if the patient's weight shows signs of increasing at some point in the future. It should also be explained that it is best to prepare in advance for such times rather than hope that they will never occur. Patients should be reminded that although they may at the moment be very aware of what has helped them, if their weight starts to creep up in 5 years' time they may be glad to have a detailed reminder of all the strategies and procedures that they found helpful so that they can reintroduce elements that they may have forgotten or neglected.

As homework, patients should be asked to think about what their written weight maintenance plan might usefully contain. It should be made clear that there are no "right answers," and that the important thing is to consider what will be most helpful for them individually. The "Draft Maintenance Plan" handout (Table 11.1; Handout V) provides commonly used headings to help patients think about the subject.

Therapists should also suggest that patients consider the various components of treatment and note down which worked best. With regard to those elements that were not helpful, patients should consider whether this was because they

TABLE 11.1

Draft Maintenance Plan

DRAFT MAINTENANCE PLAN

Make some notes under the following headings.

1. Reasons I do not want to regain weight:
    a.
    b.
    c.
    d.
2. Good habits to keep up (eating):
    a.
    b.
    c.
    d.
3. Good habits to keep up (activity):
    a.
    b.
    c.
    d.
4. Danger areas to be aware of:
    a.
    b.
    c.
    d.

---

were ineffective, not appropriate, or improperly implemented. If these elements might be useful now, or at some point in the future, they should also be noted.

Finally, patients should also be encouraged to note what situations might be likely to lead them to gain weight in the future, and how they should envisage dealing with them.

Step 2

Using the patient's completed homework as a starting point, the therapist and patient should collaboratively draft a weight maintenance plan and, before the final session, the therapist should prepare a written version for the patient to keep. An example plan is shown in Table 11.2.

Step 3

Therapists should give patients the written weight maintenance plan and review it with them. Patients should be asked to suggest additions or amendments, and they should subsequently be sent (or given there and then) a completed version of the maintenance plan.

TABLE 11.2

An Example Maintenance Plan

MY WEIGHT MAINTENANCE PLAN

This document is important. I will always be prone to gain weight. It will help me minimize the problem. I need to reread it at regular intervals. Each time, I will write in my diary a reminder of the next time I should reread this plan.

Reasons I do not want to gain weight

It is important to remember why I do not want to gain weight:
- I feel much fitter now.
- I have more energy.
- I am not excluded from things because of my weight now. I can get up stairs easily, and I can keep up with other people.
- Clothes are no longer the issue they were.
- I feel that I no longer stand out from other people because of my size.
- I no longer think "I cannot do what other people can do."

Weight maintenance

1. My goal weight range

My goal weight range is 200–208 lb. I will try to stay within the tramlines during the next 6 months as I need to practice maintaining my weight. After that, if I consider trying to lose more weight, I will first ask myself why I want to lose weight. I will ensure that I am being realistic. I will think about the pros and cons, remembering that it is harder to maintain a lower weight. I will remind myself that it is much better for me to learn to successfully maintain this weight than to try to lose a few more pounds and risk regaining weight. I will think about whether it is a good time to try to lose weight.

If I do decide to try to lose more weight, I will do so in a manner that is in keeping with this treatment (rather than trying "fad diets"). I will set myself a clearly defined time to try to lose weight (e.g., 3 months), and I will review my progress at monthly intervals. After the 3 months (or in less time if I have got as far as I can or want to), I will resume weight maintenance in order to "lock onto" my new weight.

2. Good habits (eating)

I want to keep up these good habits:
- Remaining aware of what I eat
- Eating three meals a day
- Not eating too much (e.g., generally not having seconds)
- Not eating too fast (especially when stressed)
- Not eating too often (e.g., not too many snacks)
- But not having too long a gap without eating either
- Planning ahead and taking lunch with me to work
- Limiting the amount of alcohol I drink (e.g., by having some alcohol-free days), and reminding myself that I feel better when I have not drunk much alcohol
- Choosing low-fat varieties of food
- Eating plenty of fruit and vegetables (aiming for at least five portions per day)
- Eating bread, cereal, rice, or pasta at each meal
- Not eating food straight out of the package
- Chewing sugar-free gum if I want to chew something while in the car
- Checking the calories of new foods if I'm not sure about them and comparing brands when I'm shopping

continued

TABLE 11.2

(continued)

- Throwing leftovers away or giving them to a friend
- Leaving some food on the plate when I eat out
- Compensating by eating less on other days if I have eaten more one day
- Occasionally weighing food, to check that my portions have not got bigger
- Not having any "banned foods," but letting myself have a small amount of something if I want it, while being careful not to eat too much over all
- "Urge surfing" when I am tempted to eat at a time when I am not really hungry

3. Good habits (activity)

I want to keep active by:
- Reminding myself of the benefits of being active
- Cycling
- Walking as much as I can

4. Danger areas

1. I am prone to turn to food when I feel under stress. This increases my risk of weight gain, and it does not ease the stress. I will try to use other ways to cope with problems that help me feel better in the longer term. I will also face problems and use problem solving to find solutions.
2. I have a tendency to neglect my achievements. I will also try not to confuse "feeling low" with "feeling fat."
3. Sometimes I have overeaten because I felt tired. I will try to look after myself and ensure that I make enough time to relax and rest, so that I do not feel exhausted.
4. In the past I have tended to think in "black-and-white" terms. Now I know that no food is "forbidden." If I have overeaten or gained some weight, I can talk myself through the difficulties and get back on track right away.
5. Another danger area can be when I am feeding other people. I must remember that I do not have to prepare high-calorie food for other people. I have also learned that I do not have to invite people for meals at all unless I want to! If I do invite people over, I will try to enjoy the occasion as a whole and not overeat.

5. Weight monitoring and reviewing

I will need to continue weighing myself indefinitely because I will always be at risk of gaining weight. It is better to accept the problem than pretend it is not there. *I must beware of not weighing myself. I will weigh myself every Friday morning, and I will plot this weight* on my weight graph to look for signs of weight change.

6. When to act

I must take action if any of the following occur:

1. If my weight crosses the tramlines (moving outside the 200- to 208-lb range)
2. If there is evidence of steady weight gain over 4 weeks
3. If there has been a sudden change (4 lb or more) in my weight

If my weight has been rising but is still inside the tramlines, I will make a deliberate effort to be especially careful about what I eat. It is important that I do this, because it is much easier to nip the problem in the bud than to lose weight after it has risen further. If my weight has gone above the tramlines, I will need to consider the following issues:

continued

TABLE 11.2

Dealing with setbacks

1. Evaluating the change in weight

- Is it a sudden leap or a gradual trend?

2. Identifying the cause(s)

There are three potential causes:

1. A change in food intake—the most likely
2. A change in activity
3. Ill health

I will collect information to work out what has caused the weight gain, and I will resume monitoring. This will involve calorie counting (and, therefore, weighing food). I have learned that likely causes of my gaining weight are an increase in portion sizes, poor food choice, and stress-related eating. I will also think about my level of activity. Am I spending too much time sitting down? Am I still being active during the day and going to the gym?

3. Identifying the background cause(s)

I will have to think about what else is going on that might be leading me to gain weight. I will need to think about my life over the past few months. Have there been any relevant changes? Am I under stress? Or have my habits just deteriorated?

4. Devising a plan for dealing with the change in weight

- *Stage 1.* I will need to establish an energy deficit to bring my weight back into the middle of the tramlines. This will generally involve cutting back on food intake for some weeks (to, say, 1,500 calories). I will need to regularly evaluate my progress (about every 3 days) and adjust my plans accordingly.
- *Stage 2.* Once my weight is about right, I will need to make further adjustments to my eating to stabilize my weight. I will also need to tackle the changes in my eating and activity that led to my weight gain. At some point I will need to stop recording my food intake.

5. Devising a plan for dealing with the background cause(s)

If there is a background problem, I will use the problem-solving approach to tackle it. I will need to regularly review my progress.

Ending Treatment

At the final treatment session, therapists should congratulate patients on their achievements, and ask how they feel about treatment as a whole and about the fact that treatment is to end. Any remaining issues should again be addressed. Patients should be encouraged to occasionally reread the weight maintenance plan, especially if their weight is showing signs of rising. They should also be reminded to continue weighing themselves once a week and recording their weight on their graph. It is our practice to provide a supply of about 20 blank weight graphs as a tangible sign that they are expected to continue filling them in. The top copy should be tailored to the individual patient highlighting the patient's initial weight (if the patient has lost a substantial amount of weight), and marking out the agreed tramlines.

Therapists should do their best to ensure that treatment always ends in a positive manner, with the therapist conveying the expectation that the patient will continue to follow the guidelines that have proved useful in treatment. Patients should be reminded that they have learned how to deal effectively with weight gain, and that if they follow these guidelines, they should be protected against regaining the weight that they have lost.

It is good practice to offer patients several follow-up appointments after the end of treatment.[4] We suggest that these be held at about 2-month intervals. They may be viewed as "booster sessions," providing patients with an opportunity to check in and discuss any problems that might be arising.

[4]Although this is our general recommendation, it was not our practice in the Oxford study. This is because our aim was to see whether the treatment alone, without subsequent support, would be superior to more conventional methods of weight control.

Patient Handouts

RECORDING YOUR EATING

The importance of recording cannot be stressed too much. It is vital if treatment is to succeed. Recording will help you identify exactly which aspects of your behavior you need to change, *and it will help you make these changes.*

At this stage you need to record everything that you eat and drink. A simple description will do. To do this, you will need to carry your records with you. The following instructions are to help you complete the records.

- Column 1 is for noting the exact time of day you ate or drank the items concerned. You should write things down as soon as possible afterward.
- Column 2 is for giving a simple description of what was eaten and drunk. You should record absolutely everything consumed. Please identify meals with brackets.
- Column 3 is for noting where you were at the time. If at home, please note the room.
- An asterisk should be placed in column 4 beside anything you ate or drank that you viewed as excessive. This should be your view not other people's.
- Column 5 is for noting calories.
- Column 6 is for noting other points of relevance (e.g., your thoughts or feelings, the circumstances, or context in which the eating occurred). You should also note your weight in this column each time that you weigh yourself.

Please remember to bring your records to each treatment session.

EXAMPLE FOOD DIARY

DAY Wednesday   DATE 7th October

Time	Food and Drink Consumed	Place	*	Calories	Comments
8.45 am	2 slices brown bread	kitchen	*	160	Did not really
	14g butter		*	102	want it
	14g peanut butter		*	87	Eating without
	water			0	thinking.
8.55					Weight 103kg Too heavy.
10.50	Diet coke	work			
12.50	Chocolate from vending machine	work	*	255	Calories on pack. I had planned to go to canteen, but 4 people I knew were there and I didn't want them to see me eat.
1p.m.	prawn mayonnaise sandwich (low fat)	In town		283	Calories on pack
	diet coke			0	
	chocolate bar		*	255	Did not want it, do not know why I ate it.
15.00	Diet coke	work		0	
18.05	1 gin and tonic	pub		85	Out with colleagues. Did not enjoy it – I was thinking about my food problems
19.40	Half a loaf of bread (i.e. 400g)	dining room	*	880	I estimated calories as I did not weigh it. I feel awful. I cannot believe I've done this again.
	butter		*	510	
	peanut butter		*	435	
	4 glasses red wine		*	340	
		TOTAL		3392	I'm going to bed.

EXAMPLE FOOD DIARY

DAY ...Sunday.............   DATE...... 15th August...

Time	Food and Drink Consumed	Place	*	Calories	Comments
10 a.m.	2 slices toast	front room		158	
	cream cheese (light)			25	
	black coffee			0	
11.40 am	10 Pringles	front room		110	Saw them and could not resist!
Noon	nectarine	kitchen		80	Think I was just bored.
1.40	2 slices toast	front room		158	
	cream cheese (light)			25	
	diet coke			0	
6.30	chicken (9oz)	front room		306	Very satisfying meal
	roast potatoes (4oz)			172	
	carrots (8oz)			80	
	cauliflower (9oz)			90	
7.20	large orange (13oz)	kitchen		91	
9pm	medium banana	friend's house		114	I couldn't weigh this, so calories are an estimate.
9.40	glass of wine (medium, white)	friend's house		95	
		TOTAL		1504	I'm pleased with today

A BLANK MONITORING RECORD

DAY:			DATE:		
Time	Food and Drink Consumed	Place	*	Calories	Comments

ENERGY BALANCE

The key points

- To have a stable weight, your energy intake (what you eat as food and drink) must equal the energy you burn up (that needed to keep your body processes going and for physical activity).

- Weight problems develop when your energy intake (calories) exceeds the energy you are burning up over a sustained period of time.

- This positive energy balance (excess energy) is stored in the body mainly as fat.

- Excess weight (fat) is only lost when you create a negative energy balance so that your body draws on its energy (fat) stores.

- A sustained reduction in your energy intake (as food and drink) is needed to produce weight loss.

- In principle your rate of weight loss could be accelerated by increasing the energy you burn up as a result of physical activity, but in practice the additional benefits are not great. On the other hand, regular physical activity does help weight maintenance.

- Once you reach your target weight range, you will need to adjust your eating and activity level to stabilize your weight. This is an important skill that requires practice.

Why do some people develop weight problems?

- There are two main reasons and often they both apply:

  - Eating too much (energy intake too high)

  - Not being active enough (not burning enough energy)

- Metabolic, hormonal, or other medical problems are rarely relevant, although people vary somewhat in the amount of energy their body needs to keep running.

- Weight problems tend to run in families. This can be due to the family environment or to genetic factors or both.

- Genes have a definite influence on body weight, so if you come from a family in which many people have significant weight problems, you are likely to be genetically vulnerable to similar difficulties.

- Psychological factors lead some people to overeat. Some people overeat in response to stress or when they are unhappy or bored, whereas others find that their appetite is diminished. Extreme dieting can also encourage overeating.

- Poor eating habits can also be learned (at home, school or work, or due to other circumstances). A particular problem in our society today is that most people eat too much high-fat food, largely because it is readily available and tastes good.

- As a society we are also much less active than we used to be. Many people have jobs that involve little activity and people are also much less active at home.

REVIEW SESSIONS

Now that your appointments will be at 2-week intervals, it is important to have weekly, between-session, appointments with yourself. This might seem odd but it can be extremely valuable. The purpose of these review sessions is to ensure that you remain alert to your progress and any problems that you might be having. They also help you maintain momentum between our sessions.

These review sessions are important and should be given priority. It is best to schedule them in advance just like a treatment appointment. It is helpful if each session has the following structure:

- Review of your progress based on your most recent monitoring records and any change in your weight. In doing this you should take account of the "homework" that was agreed at the last session.
- Identify everything that you have achieved over the last week. It is important to give yourself credit for your achievements.
- Set yourself one or two specific goals for the forthcoming week.

It is also very important to continue to weigh yourself at weekly intervals and record your weight on your graph.

At each appointment we will discuss how you have managed with the review and the goals that you set yourself.

Making a habit of assessing your progress in this way will prepare you for the future when you will no longer be coming for treatment.

SOCIAL EATING

Eating out or with other people can pose additional challenges when you are trying to control your calorie intake. Planning ahead is important. In particular, it is helpful to ensure that you have thought about how to deal with both the practical issues related to social eating and your attitude to keeping to your calorie limit. Most situations can be successfully tackled if you have a plan for dealing with them. On the other hand, if you are caught unawares you are at greater risk of experiencing problems.

Here are some specific tips for dealing with eating out.

A. Practical Strategies

General

- Plan far enough in advance, as you may want to adjust your eating in the days before (and/or after) the event to "bank" calories. You will often also need to plan a strategy to deal with the specific situation (see below).
- Think about the difficulties you will encounter. Consider the following:
  - The amounts and types of food that will be provided
  - Social pressures to eat
  - The availability of "extras" (e.g., premeal appetizers, after-dinner chocolates)
  - Alcohol
- It may be useful to think about how you have dealt with similar situations in the past.

In all the situations mentioned below it is helpful to plan in advance. This gives you time to anticipate any difficulties that might arise and how to cope with them. Here are some practical tips that may help. Note that not all will suit you or the situation.

Restaurants

- Participate in the choice of restaurant if possible; look at the menu in advance, or possibly telephone the restaurant to ask about availability of low-fat or low-calorie dishes.
- If possible, ask for food to be served without extra butter, and for dressings and sauces to be served separately so you can control the amount you have. Consider asking for a smaller portion of the main dish with extra vegetables or salad.
- Be wary of set menus. They may include dishes that are not good choices for people who are trying to lose weight, but are also difficult to resist when you have already paid for them.
- Try asking for fresh fruit as a dessert, or maybe share a dessert with somebody else.

continued

Buffets

- Look carefully at what is available before you actually put anything on your plate. Identify a few foods that you would really enjoy (rather than trying a bit of everything) and choose some low-calorie options such as salad or rice to fill you up.

- Try using a side plate rather than a full-size dinner plate.

- Treat it as you would a sit-down meal. Visit the buffet table only once, and then when you have eaten get rid of your plate as soon as possible.

- Alternatively, ask someone else to bring you some food, and tell them what you would like.

Entertaining in Your Own Home

- Consider whether you are obliged to provide a high-fat, high-calorie meal. Many people are either watching their weight or being careful about their diet for health reasons. A lower-fat meal is just as likely to be welcomed by guests and certainly does not indicate poor hospitality.

- Single-portion foods, such as individual chicken pieces, are often easier to manage and avoid the difficulty of having tempting leftovers.

- If you do have food left over, either give it to guests to take with them or freeze it immediately.

- If you tend to pick while preparing food, try immersing used dishes and utensils immediately in soapy water or chewing gum while you cook.

Eating at Someone Else's House

- If possible, try to find out in advance what will be served. If you know the host/hostess well, consider contacting them in advance to explain your situation and ask if it would be possible for him or her to help. You could perhaps find out what he or she is planning to serve so that you can decide in advance what you will eat, and plan your day accordingly.

- It may be possible to offer to take a dish with you, so that you know there will be at least one low-calorie option.

- Offer to help serve so that you can control your portion size, or ask for a small portion.

- Fill your plate with salad or vegetables, and take only small amounts of high-calorie dishes. This helps to control the calories and avoids drawing attention to your weight control efforts.

- Asking for recipes may be a good (and socially acceptable) way of finding out what went into a meal so as to calculate the calories you consumed.

continued

B. Other Issues

Pressure to Eat

If you tend to feel under pressure to eat more than you had planned, try to work out exactly what makes you feel this way. Are you concerned that people will be offended if you do not eat everything you are offered, or that you will draw attention to yourself if you do not eat as much as everyone else? If you can work out precisely what the problem is, it will be easier to think of ways to cope. For example, if you are concerned that your host will be offended if you do not eat much, you might decide it would be helpful to practice saying "No" politely but firmly. You could test out whether politely declining foods is likely to cause offence. You might do this by thinking about how you would feel if you were the host and someone declined food in this way; or by watching carefully to see if other people always eat large portions of everything available, and how others react if they do not. If you are concerned about drawing attention to yourself by not doing what everyone else is doing, you might observe the reactions of others to people who, for example, are not drinking alcohol, perhaps because they are driving, or perhaps simply because it is their preference not to do so. Ask yourself whether you think it would be reasonable to react negatively to such situations and whether you would do so.

Feeling Deprived

Although planning ahead to make the most of your calories is helpful, it is not uncommon to feel that social events revolve entirely around high-calorie food and drink and to think that not being able to eat or drink everything that you would like will make these events less enjoyable. You could test this view to see whether you really enjoy occasions less if you limit your food and alcohol. Also, you could try focusing on all those nonfood aspects of social events that make them enjoyable (e.g., talking to friends, having time to relax, not having to wash the dishes) so that food and drink become less important aspects of social events.

Coping with Unexpected Occasions

Sometimes invitations to eat arrive unexpectedly—someone drops in and suggests having lunch together, or friends come around with take-out, or somebody suggests going for a meal after a movie. It is helpful to take a few minutes to think clearly about how to handle the situation. You may decide to join in with the meal, and cut down on calories later in the day or the next day. Alternatively, if you have already eaten or planned what you are going to eat, you may need to respond differently: perhaps by suggesting another time when you could have a meal together or explaining that you will just have a small amount as you have already eaten. You may wish to experiment with different possibilities and find out which one works best for you.

PLANNING FOR VACATIONS

Vacations can pose additional challenges when you are trying to control your calorie intake. You may be in unfamiliar surroundings where the food choice may be quite different from home, and you may have less control than usual over the preparation of food.

Planning ahead is important. In particular, it is helpful to ensure that you have thought about how to deal with both the practical issues related to eating, as well as how you might feel about keeping to a calorie limit. Most situations can be successfully tackled if you have a plan for dealing with them. On the other hand, if you are caught unawares you are at greater risk of encountering problems.

General

Vacations are a time to relax and enjoy yourself, and sometimes people see this as incompatible with restricting their consumption of food and drink. It is worth considering how you can make the most of your vacation without undoing all the hard work you have put into losing weight. The first step is to decide on your goal over the vacation. Do you want to continue losing weight or to maintain your current weight? If you intend to stick to your calorie goal with the aim of continuing to lose weight, be clear and realistic about how you will achieve this goal. If you think that it is not realistic to stick to your calorie goal, it may be best to work out a slightly higher calorie limit with your therapist for the vacation period, with the aim of maintaining your weight.

In making decisions about your goals, it may be helpful to consider what, besides being able to drink and eat freely, will be enjoyable about the time away. A vacation may provide an ideal opportunity to practice the new habits you have learned and experiment with the possibility that you can have an enjoyable time while still limiting your intake of food and alcohol.

Here are some specific practical issues to consider when planning ahead.

Monitoring Food and Weight

- Will you monitor your food and weight while you are away? If so, how? Will scales be available for weighing food and for checking your weight?

- When will you do your weekly reviews? Can you set aside a time with yourself? Would it be helpful to send (fax or E-mail) your weekly reviews to your therapist while you are away?

continued

Arrangements for Travel

- How long will your journey take from door to door? What meals would you normally eat during this time? Will you be traveling overnight or on a long-haul flight? If so, how this might affect your eating pattern?

- What food will be available? Is it worth taking your own to ensure you have control over what you eat? Are you likely to be tempted by the availability of snack foods in gas stations, airports, or trains? Will your food choice be determined by circumstances (e.g., food on an airplane)? If so, would it be worthwhile ordering a special meal?

- What time will it be when you arrive at your destination (and at home on your return journey)? Can you arrange for suitable food to be available (e.g., by leaving a meal in the freezer at home)?

- How can you make it easy to keep monitoring while you travel? Many people find it is difficult to resume monitoring after a gap, so working out how to monitor through unusual situations is worthwhile. Making sure you have your monitoring sheets handy is important, and calculating in advance anything you take with you can make monitoring easier during the journey.

General Arrangements When Away

- Will food be provided? Will you be eating out, preparing your own food, or a combination of these? How will you cope with the particular arrangements? Do you anticipate any difficulties? Planning ahead is likely to be helpful in these situations.

- How will your requirements fit in with the rest of the party?

- What types of food will be available?

Alcohol

- Does your alcohol intake tend to increase when on vacation? How do you intend to manage this?

SPECIAL OCCASIONS

Controlling your calorie intake on special occasions (such as parties, birthdays, weddings, and other celebrations) can be difficult. Such occasions provide a good opportunity to practice the new habits you are learning and to experiment with the possibility of having an enjoyable time without eating too much. This handout summarizes many of the strategies that we recommend for coping with special occasions. It also suggests new and different ways to think about the role of food on special occasions.

Goals

It is generally best to stick to your usual weekly calorie goal (as an average over the week). Be clear and realistic about how you will achieve this. Eating nothing all day in anticipation of a party is likely to lead to overeating later on. Instead, eating lightly the day before or after may be a better plan. Completely avoiding food that you like may also be a mistake. It is usually a good idea to plan to eat such food and incorporate it into your day's eating plan.

Plan Ahead

The single most important strategy for dealing with any special occasion is planning ahead. This is especially important if there will be extra food around over a period of several days, and if there will be more than one special meal or party. High-calorie foods and alcoholic drinks often seem to be an integral part of these events, so it is especially important that you make plans to deal with these challenges. It is generally helpful to make a plan for each day, and you may need to plan several days in advance when celebrations go on for several days.

Monitor

It is very important to continue to monitor. This will keep you informed about how your strategies are working and help you to adjust your plans as necessary. It will also help you to keep focused on your goals.

Alcohol

It is especially important to have a plan for dealing with alcohol; not only does it add calories, but it tends to weaken the resolve to eat moderately.

Focus on Other Pleasurable Aspects of Special Occasions

Although many social events may seem to center on high-calorie food and drinks, consider whether it is possible to celebrate without consuming these in large quantities. It

continued

may be helpful to think about ways of making celebrations enjoyable that do not involve eating (or at least eating large quantities of food) and trying these out. Try paying particular attention to the features of social occasions that make them enjoyable. This may lead you to conclude that eating moderate quantities of food would not spoil your enjoyment. Some people even discover that they enjoy occasions more when they eat and drink less.

Dealing with Pressure to Eat

You may feel under pressure to eat more than you had planned. This can happen for many reasons: The sheer abundance of food may tempt you; you may feel people will be offended if you do not eat much; or you may feel that you will be 'the odd one out' if you do not join others in eating and drinking all that is offered. It is always easier to cope with such situations if you have made a plan in advance. Also it is helpful to practice refusing food politely but firmly. You do not have to eat to please others, and people rarely notice what you are eating and drinking.

Gifts of Food

On special occasions people may buy chocolate, sweets, cake, or other food for you. If this is likely, would it be worth asking them to buy something else instead? If you feel you could not make this request yourself, perhaps your partner or a relative or friend could discreetly advise others that you would prefer not to be given food. Also it would be helpful to consider how to cope if you receive such food unexpectedly. Could you give it to someone else?

Snacks

Sometimes on special occasions there is a wide variety of snacks on display. Having bowls of nuts, chocolates, and other high-calorie snacks is likely to be a temptation beyond most people's endurance, so plan how best to cope with this situation. When such situations are under your control, you may decide to do things differently.

If you are having to provide snacks:

- Plan the shopping carefully and limit the amount of extra food bought.
- Keep snacks in sealed containers, and only set out small quantities for specific occasions.
- Have alternative, lower-calorie snacks such as raw vegetables with low-calorie dip, fruit, plain (unsweetened or unbuttered) popcorn, and bread sticks.
- The strategies suggested in Handout G on social eating are also relevant to many special occasions.

PROBLEM SOLVING

As discussed in the session, effective problem solving involves six basic steps together with a final review step. The six steps are as follows:

Step 1. Identify the problem as early as possible.

Step 2. Specify the problem accurately.

Step 3. Consider as many solutions as possible.

Step 4. Think through the implications of each solution.

Step 5. Choose the best solution or combination of solutions.

Step 6. Act on the solution.

Then, afterward, review the whole problem-solving process to see if you could have done it any better. You will improve with practice.

BARRIERS TO WEIGHT LOSS CHECKLIST

Below is a list of commonly encountered barriers to weight loss. Please consider which (if any) apply to you, and place a tick in the relevant column.

	No	To some extent	Yes
Accuracy of recording:			
Is absolutely everything written down?			
Do you accurately measure your portions?			
Do you carefully calculate calories?			
Weighing and weekly reviews:			
Are you weighing yourself once a week?			
Are you holding weekly review sessions?			
Your eating pattern (i.e., when you eat):			
Do your eating habits vary greatly from day to day?			
Do you eat regular meals and snacks through the day?			
Do you skip any meals?			
Do you go for long periods without eating?			
Do you tend to nibble or pick at food?			
Are there particular times of day (or particular days) when you are liable to overeat?			
Do you have "binges" (large or small)?			
Your portion sizes:			
Are your portion sizes on the large side?			
Do you take second helpings?			
Do you always "clean your plate"?			
Do you eat leftovers?			
Your choice of foods and drink:			
Are you prone to eat energy-rich (i.e., high-fat) foods?			
Are you actively avoiding any foods?			

continued

	No	To some extent	Yes
How you eat:			
Are you someone who eats very rapidly?	_____	_____	_____
Do you eat in places other than the kitchen or dining room?	_____	_____	_____
Do you eat while watching television?	_____	_____	_____
Do you eat while driving or engaged in other activities?	_____	_____	_____
Is your eating planned in advance?	_____	_____	_____
Do you eat directly from packets or containers?	_____	_____	_____
Other obstacles to weight loss:			
Have you lost your motivation to lose weight?	_____	_____	_____
Are you prone to stress-related eating?	_____	_____	_____
Are you liable to eat when bored?	_____	_____	_____
Does thinking in black-and-white terms undermine your attempts to lose weight?	_____	_____	_____
Are you facing other obstacles to losing weight?	_____	_____	_____

MONITORING YOUR LEVEL OF ACTIVITY

The first step in increasing your level of physical activity is to measure how active you are now. To do this you need to measure the three forms of activity discussed in treatment.

Inactivity

At the end of each day recall as accurately as you can how many hours you have spent sitting or lying down. Do this for a 24-hour period (midnight to midnight) projecting forward for the few hours remaining in the day. Then record the number in an "activity box" drawn on the back of the day's monitoring record (see below). If you sit down at work, it may be best to keep a running total of the time spent sitting in column 6 of your monitoring record.

Lifestyle Activity

This term refers to incidental physical activities that are part of day-to-day life. It includes walking, standing, climbing stairs, household chores, light gardening, ordinary cycling, and gentle swimming.

With the exception of cycling and swimming, we recommend quantifying these activities in an approximate way (in terms of the number of steps taken) using a pedometer.

If you have a pedometer, you should wear the pedometer at all times except when in bed and engaging in formal exercise (see below). You should put it on first thing in the morning. To remember to do this, attach it to something you use first thing in the morning (e.g., a comb or hair brush) and return the reading to zero by pressing the reset button. Attach the pedometer to a belt or article of clothing at the side of your hips. Then, last thing at night, note the number of steps recorded in the day's activity box. Please note that you should ignore any calorie table that may come with the pedometer as such figures are generally misleading.

Formal Exercise

At the end of each day you should also record in the activity box the number of minutes spent engaged in formal exercise. To be classed as formal exercise, the exercise should involve exertion to the point that your pulse and breathing rate are increased. Such exercise includes jogging, moderate-to-fast swimming, brisk walking, and fast cycling.

continued

Activity Box

The activity box summarizes your level of activity over the previous 24 hours. It should be drawn on the back of the day's monitoring record and completed at the end of the day. It should look like this:

Inactivity (hours)	8 hours in bed, 3 hours sitting
Lifestyle activity (steps)	3,860 steps
Formal exercise (minutes and type)	None today

THE BODY IMAGE CHECKLIST

Instructions: Please answer these questions as they have applied to you over the PAST 4 WEEKS. Please place a tick in the appropriate column.

Over the past 4 weeks ...	Not at all	Sometimes	Frequently	Not applicable
Questions about avoidance:				
Have you avoided seeing yourself in mirrors (or window reflections)?				
Have you avoided weighing yourself?				
Have you dressed in a way to disguise your appearance?				
Have you avoided your shape being seen by others (e.g., swimming pools, communal changing rooms, etc.)?				
Have you avoided taking part in physical activities because of your shape?				
Have you avoided shopping for clothes?				
Have you avoided being seen at home naked (e.g., when undressing or bathing)?				
Have you avoided wearing clothes that show the shape of your body?				
Have you avoided (or limited) close physical contact because of your dislike of your shape (e.g., shaking hands, sexual contact, hugging, kissing)?				
Have you avoided wearing clothes that show your skin (e.g., short-sleeve shirts, shorts)?				
Have you avoided social occasions because of your shape?				
Questions about checking:				
Have you studied your overall appearance in the mirror?				
Have you studied parts of your body in the mirror?				
Have you weighed yourself?				

continued

Over the past 4 weeks ...	Not at all	Sometimes	Frequently	Not applicable
Have you measured parts of your body?	_____	_____	_____	_____
Have you assessed your size in other ways?	_____	_____	_____	_____
Have you pinched yourself to see how much fat there is?	_____	_____	_____	_____
General questions:	_____	_____	_____	_____
Have you felt unhappy about your shape?	_____	_____	_____	_____
Have you worried about the size of particular parts of your body?	_____	_____	_____	_____
Have you worried about your body wobbling?	_____	_____	_____	_____
Have you felt ashamed or embarrassed about your body in public?	_____	_____	_____	_____
Have you felt that other people were noticing your shape?	_____	_____	_____	_____
Have you felt that your body was disgusting?	_____	_____	_____	_____
Have you thought that other people were being critical of you because of your shape?	_____	_____	_____	_____
Have you felt that you take up too much room (e.g., when sitting on a sofa or bus seat)?	_____	_____	_____	_____
Have you sought reassurance that your shape is not as bad as you think it is?	_____	_____	_____	_____
Have people made critical comments about your shape or appearance?	_____	_____	_____	_____

A BLANK BODY IMAGE DIARY

Record on the body image diary times when: you were thinking negatively about your body; you avoided situations because of the way you felt about your body; you were checking your body in an inappropriate way.

Situation	Feelings	Thoughts	Behavior	Consequences	Alternative thoughts

A COMPLETED BODY IMAGE DIARY—EXAMPLE I: AVOIDANCE

Record on the body image diary times when: you were thinking negatively about your body; you were feeling upset because of the way you felt about your body; you avoided situations because of the way you felt about your body; you were checking your body in an inappropriate way.

Situation	Feelings	Thoughts	Behavior	Consequences	Alternative thoughts
Being asked by my child to accompany him on a bike ride.	Anxious about what to say, sad and miserable about the situation.	The whole street will see me looking ridiculous on a bicycle. I will wobble. I cannot ride my bike until my body looks better. This is another thing I cannot do because of the way I look.	Told my son that I could not go. Made up an excuse (lied).	Not able to do things with my son, always putting things off until I get thinner.	It is me who thinks I will look ridiculous and disgusting. I am assuming everyone will think this; I do not actually know what everyone thinks. In the past I have been surprised that people have not always been thinking what I thought they were—in this case perhaps I could find out. If I saw someone who was overweight riding a bicycle I would not think they looked ridiculous—I would think it was healthy exercise. So why do I have to wait until I lose weight? Other people seem to be able to do it who are even heavier than me. Besides, I used to enjoy riding a bicycle, and it is good exercise. By saying I cannot do it, I will deprive myself of the opportunity of doing exercise that might make me feel better about myself. I should try to ride and find out what happens.

A COMPLETED BODY IMAGE DIARY—EXAMPLE 2: REPEATED CHECKING

Record on the body image diary times when: you were thinking negatively about your body; you avoided situations because of the way you felt about your body; you were checking your body in an inappropriate way.

Situation	Feelings	Thoughts	Behavior	Consequences	Alternative thoughts
Getting dressed in the morning.	Really miserable, disgusted and angry with myself.	My hips and bottom are so big. I do not look nice in these clothes—in fact nothing looks good on me. I always look terrible.	I try on several outfits in the hope that they will hide my hips and bottom. I check myself in the mirror several times and from all angles to see if I look any better. I eventually choose an outfit that is slightly better, but not much.	Once again, I'm late for work because it takes so long to dress, and I still spend all day worrying about how I look. I repeatedly go to the restroom to check myself in the mirror—still don't like what I see. When I buy clothes, I only consider whether they will hide my hips and bottom— I don't bother considering anything else.	Rationally, I know my shape cannot really have changed noticeably overnight. I felt OK at work yesterday, so the fact that I feel low today is not because I am fatter, but because I am upset about something else. My colleagues are not going to be watching me to see if my shape has changed overnight, but they will notice if I'm late for work. I know that anyone who scrutinizes themselves in a mirror could find things about their appearance that they want to change. Constantly examining myself in the mirror just makes me feel worse especially as I only look at the bits I hate— I don't bother about my hair and eyes, which are OK. So I will try to stop doing that. I am doing what I can to help myself—I have already lost some weight, although it has been slower than I would like. Now I will just make the best of where I am at the moment. I may try buying some new clothes that I feel really good in.

A COMPLETED BODY IMAGE DIARY—EXAMPLE 3: NEGATIVE THOUGHTS

Record on the body image diary times when: you were thinking negatively about your body; you avoided situations because of the way you felt about your body; you were checking your body in an inappropriate way.

Situation	Feelings	Thoughts	Behavior	Consequences	Alternative thoughts
Sitting in dentist's waiting room looking at clothes in a fashion magazine.	Envious of models looking good in great clothes, miserable and disgusted with my body.	I never look good in clothes. I cannot fit into any decent clothes any way. It is not fair; the women in the magazine are so thin and attractive, and my body is so fat and ugly.	Felt so bad I bought a bar of chocolate on the way home to console myself.	Felt even worse later because eating chocolate will make me even fatter and make the situation worse.	Just because I am not thin and perfect like a model does not mean that I am unattractive. I know people whom I regard as attractive and they don't look like models. I am comparing myself to an ideal no one can attain—photographs of models are touched up to remove imperfections.

I always compare myself to people whom I think are more attractive than I am, and not to those who are less attractive. If someone else did that, I would think they were being unfair. Perhaps I am being unduly hard on myself because I never think of the things I am good at. I know that society's ideals for shape are narrow, and I admire people who are not so influenced by them. Thinking the way I do is not helpful, because it results in my eating the wrong things, which only makes things worse.

Although I weigh more than I would like to, this does not mean that I am totally unattractive or that I cannot look stylish. |

YOUR WEIGHT GOALS

We have begun to discuss your weight goals. As "homework" we would like you to set aside some time before the next session to consider the issues listed below. We suggest you write out your answers (perhaps in note form).

You will remember that we discussed your "desired" weight, the weight that you think that you really ought to achieve. Please answer the following questions with reference to your desired weight. Please answer them in this order.

1. Origins of your desired weight:
   - Why do you want to be this specific weight?
   - Is there anything particularly special about this weight?

2. Other weight goals in the past:
   - Have you had other weight goals in the past?
   - Why were they different from your present goal?

3. Achievability of your desired weight:
   - When were you last at your desired weight?
   - How hard do you think it would be to stay at this weight?

4. Importance of reaching your desired weight:
   - How important to you is reaching your desired weight?
   - If it is important, why is it important?

5. Consequences of reaching your desired weight:
   - How would your life differ if you reached your desired weight?
   - What could you do that you cannot do now?

Or, if you have previously been this weight, How was your life different when you were at this weight?

When answering the two parts of question 5 consider the following eight aspects of daily life:

Attractiveness (to yourself and others)	Clothes size and choice
Leisure activities (e.g., sports)	Health and fitness
Work	Social life
Self-esteem and self-confidence	Personal relationships

6. Consequences of not reaching your desired weight:
   - How would you feel if you did not reach your desired weight?
   - What effect would it have on your daily life?

PLEASE REMEMBER TO BRING YOUR ANSWERS TO YOUR NEXT SESSION.

ACCEPTANCE AND CHANGE—VERSION 1

- Some aspects of the problem of being overweight can be changed; some cannot.
- A good treatment should help people change what can be changed and accept what cannot.
- Body weight is, to an important extent, genetically determined, and it is therefore only partially under one's control.
- It is possible to make fairly dramatic short-term changes in weight by severely cutting down food intake, but a great deal of research has shown that such changes cannot be sustained in the long term.
- There is currently no treatment for being overweight (other than gastrointestinal surgery) that results in a weight loss of more than 10–15% of initial body weight, and the weight lost is generally regained. Typically a third of the lost weight is regained within 1 year and almost all of it is regained within 5 years. This is true of all nonsurgical treatments (e.g., dietary treatments, very-low-calorie diets, behavior modification, and appetite suppressant drugs) as well as combinations of these treatments.
- If you lost 10–15% of your starting weight, you would weigh _____ .
- For most people, their desired weight is far lower than the weight a 10–15% loss would be. As a result they view the treatment (and/or themselves) as having failed, whereas it is really an achievement to lose this amount of weight and keep it off.
- The benefits of 10–15% weight loss can include the following:
  - Improved appearance and decrease in waist size (and therefore clothing size)
  - Enhanced sense of general well-being and self-esteem
  - Decrease in many of the negative effects on health associated with obesity (e.g., high blood pressure, high blood lipids, high blood sugar) as well as the risk of developing these problems
  - Improved sense of physical well-being
- Simultaneously treatment can address other personal goals, and generally this has a very positive effect on quality of life.

Implications for You

- You can change your weight to an important extent (10–15% weight loss), although the weight loss may well not be as great as you would wish.
- You can directly address other personal goals, but it is essential that you accept what cannot be changed (your weight range, your overall shape).

continued

- If you do not succeed in accepting what cannot be changed, you are going to be at risk of the following:
  - Undervaluing what you have achieved in treatment
  - Believing that you cannot control your weight at all
  - Not being fully committed to keeping off the weight that you have lost, a major cause of weight regain

BOTH ACCEPTANCE AND CHANGE ARE ESSENTIAL FOR SUCCESSFUL WEIGHT CONTROL.

ACCEPTANCE AND CHANGE—VERSION 2

- Some aspects of the problem of being overweight can be changed; some cannot.
- A good treatment should help people change what can be changed and accept what cannot.
- Body weight is, to an important extent, genetically determined and it is therefore only partially under one's control.
- It is possible to make fairly dramatic short-term changes in weight by severely cutting down food intake, but a great deal of research has shown that such changes cannot be sustained in the long term.
- There is currently no treatment for being overweight (other than gastrointestinal surgery) that results in a weight loss of more than 10–15% of initial body weight, and the weight lost is generally regained. Typically a third of the lost weight is regained within 1 year and almost all of it is regained within 5 years. This is true of all nonsurgical treatments (e.g., dietary treatments, very-low-calorie diets, behavior modification, and appetite suppressant drugs) as well as combinations of these treatments.
- Many people who try to lose weight do not lose as much weight as they would like to. As a result they view the treatment (and/or themselves) as having failed. In reality, it is an achievement to maintain *any* weight loss, however small. For people who have been gaining weight, to stop gaining weight is in itself an achievement.
- The benefits of 10–15% weight loss (or stopping gaining weight) can include the following:
  - Improved appearance and decrease in waist size (and therefore clothing size)
  - Enhanced sense of general well-being and self-esteem
  - Decrease in many of the negative effects on health associated with obesity (e.g., high blood pressure, high blood lipids, high blood sugar) as well as the risk of developing these problems
  - Improved sense of physical well-being
- Simultaneously treatment can address other personal goals and generally this has a very positive effect on quality of life.

Implications for You

- Although your weight loss may well not be as great as you would wish, you should see it as an achievement that you have stopped gaining weight, and have lost a certain amount of weight.

continued

- You should be aware of any other positive changes that you have made during the course of this treatment, such as addressing other personal goals.
- It is essential that you accept what cannot be changed (your weight range, your overall shape).
- If you do not succeed in accepting what cannot be changed, you are going to be at risk of the following:
  - Undervaluing what you have achieved in treatment
  - Believing that you cannot control your weight at all
  - Not being fully committed to keeping off the weight that you have lost, a major cause of weight regain

BOTH ACCEPTANCE AND CHANGE ARE ESSENTIAL FOR SUCCESSFUL WEIGHT CONTROL.

RESPONDING TO CHANGES IN WEIGHT

Each week you should inspect your weight maintenance graph, focusing on the past 4 weeks' readings. This will constitute your weekly review. This review involves:

- weighing yourself,
- plotting your latest weight on your weight maintenance graph, and
- carefully appraising the data.

If there has been a change in your weight, you will need to do the following:

1. Identify and evaluate the change in your weight.

   Questions to ask:

   - Is it a sudden leap or a gradual trend?
   - Is your body weight now outside the "tramlines"?

   Action to take:

   - Inspect your weight graph, focusing on the past four readings.

2. Identify the explanation for any change in your weight (in terms of energy intake and expenditure).

   Questions to ask:

   - Is it due to a change in eating?
   - Is it due to a change in activity?
   - Is ill health, pregnancy or medication contributing?

   Action to take:

   - To collect information, you should carefully monitor your energy intake (food and drink). Often it is wise to resume calorie counting (and, therefore, weighing food) for a while. Common causes of weight gain include an insidious increase in portion size (which often goes undetected), picking at food, a change in food choice (with increased intake of energy-dense foods), and stress-related eating.
   - You should also consider the possible role of physical activity. Have you given up certain lifestyle activities (e.g., going for walks, playing sports, going swimming)?

3. Identify the background cause(s) of any change in behavior.

   Questions to ask:

   - Is there an obvious explanation for the change?
   - Is it due to slipping into "bad habits"?

continued

Action to take:

- You should consider what factors in your life might be contributing to the change in your behavior. These are generally readily identified if there has been a recent change. More gradual changes can be more difficult to pinpoint.

4. Devise and implement a plan for addressing weight gain.

You should devise a plan for correcting the weight gain. There will need to be two phases.

- First, you will need to establish an energy deficit to bring your weight back into the middle of the tramlines. This will usually involve restricting your food intake for some weeks (to, say, 1,500 calories). You will need to closely monitor your progress (e.g., every 3 or 7 days) and adjust your strategy accordingly.
- Second, once the increase has been corrected, you will need to make further adjustments to stabilize your weight. Generally these will involve changes in both energy intake and physical activity following the guidelines which have been provided. You will also need to discontinue monitoring your food intake. You will need to continue regularly monitoring your weight.

5. Devise and implement a plan for dealing with the background cause(s) of the change in behavior.

You will also need to address the background cause. This is best done using the formal problem-solving approach. As with the changes in eating and activity, you will need to regularly evaluate your progress and adjust your plans accordingly.

DRAFT MAINTENANCE PLAN

Make some notes under the following headings.

1. Reasons I do not want to regain weight:
   a.

   b.

   c.

   d.

2. Good habits to keep up (eating):
   a.

   b.

   c.

   d.

3. Good habits to keep up (activity):
   a.

   b.

   c.

   d.

4. Danger areas to be aware of:
   a.

   b.

   c.

   d.

APPENDIX II

Useful Websites

The following table has been adapted from a similar table published in a chapter titled "Obesity and the Internet" by K. R. Fontaine and D. B. Allison from Fairburn and Brownell (2002).

Website	Description
American Dietetic Association (www.eatright.org)	Provides information on nutrition and weight control.
American Obesity Society (www.obesity.org)	Provides education for general public and health professionals and advocates for rights of obese persons.
International Obesity Task Force (www.iotf.org)	Provides education and advocacy for obesity to be viewed as a worldwide epidemic.
National Association to Advance Fat Acceptance (www.naafa.org)	Advocates on behalf of obese persons to improve quality of life and reduce discrimination.
National Heart, Lung and Blood Institute (www.nhlbi.nih.gov)	Provides resources for health professionals and the general public.
National Institute of Diabetes and Digestive and Kidney Diseases (www.niddk.nih.gov)	Provides information on weight loss and control for health professionals and the general public. Includes information about physical activity for overweight people.
North American Association for the Study of Obesity (www.naaso.org)	Interdisciplinary society that develops, extends, and disseminates knowledge in the field of obesity.
Shape Up America! (www.shapeup.org)	Provides general information on weight control and physical activity.

References

American Psychiatric Association (1994). *Diagnostic and statistical manual of mental disorders* (4th ed.). Washington, DC: Author.

Aronne, L. J. (2002). Current pharmacological treatments for obesity. In C. G. Fairburn & K. D. Brownell (Eds.), *Eating disorders and obesity: A comprehensive handbook* (2nd ed., pp. 551–556). New York: Guilford.

Beck, A. T. (1976). *Cognitive therapy and the emotional disorders.* New York: International Universities Press.

Beck, J. S. (1995). *Cognitive therapy: Basics and beyond.* New York: Guilford.

Bjorvell, H., & Rössner, S. (1992). A ten-year follow-up of weight change in severely obese subjects treated in a combined behavioural modification program. *International Journal of Obesity, 16,* 623–625.

Blackburn, G. L. (2002). Weight loss and risk factors. In C. G. Fairburn & K. D. Brownell (Eds.), *Eating disorders and obesity: A comprehensive handbook* (2nd ed., pp. 484–489). New York: Guilford.

Blair, S. N., & Holder, S. (2002). Exercise in the management of obesity. In C. G. Fairburn & K. D. Brownell (Eds.), *Eating disorders and obesity: A comprehensive handbook* (2nd ed., pp. 518–523). New York: Guilford.

Blundell, J. E. (2002). A psychobiological system approach to appetite and weight control. In C. G. Fairburn & K. D. Brownell (Eds.), *Eating disorders and obesity: A comprehensive handbook* (2nd ed., pp. 43–49). New York: Guilford.

Boutelle, K. N., & Kirschenbaum, D. S. (1998). Further support for consistent self-monitoring as a vital component of successful weight control. *Obesity Research, 6,* 219–224.

Carter, J. C., & Fairburn, C. G. (1998). Cognitive-behavioral self-help for binge eating disorder: A controlled effectiveness study. *Journal of Consulting and Clinical Psychology, 66,* 616–623.

Cash, T. F. (1994). Body image and weight changes in a multisite comprehensive very-low-calorie diet program. *Behavior Therapy, 25,* 239–254.

Cash, T. F. (1996). The treatment of body image disturbances. In J. K. Thompson (Ed.), *Body image, eating disorders, and obesity* (pp. 83–107). Washington, DC: American Psychological Association.

Cash, T. F. (1997). *The body image workbook: An 8-step program for learning to like your looks.* Oakland, CA: New Harbinger.

Cash, T. F., Counts, B., & Huffine, C. E. (1990). Current and vestigial effects of overweight among women: Fear of fat, attitudinal body image, and eating behaviors. *Journal of Psychopathology, 12,* 157–167.

Clark, D. M. (1986). A cognitive approach to panic disorder. *Behaviour Research and Therapy, 24,* 461–470.

Collins, J. K., McCabe, M. M., Jupp, J. J., & Sutton, J. E. (1983). Body percept change in obese females after weight reduction therapy. *Journal of Clinical Psychology, 39,* 507–511.

Connolly, H. M., Crary, J. L., McGoon, M. D., Hensrud, D. D., Edwards, B. S., Edwards, W. D., & Schaff, H. V. (1997). Valvular heart disease associated with fenfluramine–phentermine. *New England Journal of Medicine, 337,* 581–588.

Cooper, Z., & Fairburn, C. G. (2001). A new cognitive behavioural approach to the treatment of obesity. *Behaviour Research and Therapy, 39,* 499–511.

Cooper, Z., & Fairburn, C. G. (2002). Cognitive-behavioral treatment of obesity. In T. A. Wadden & A. J. Stunkard (Eds.), *Handbook of obesity treatment* (pp. 465–479). New York: Guilford.

DeLucia, J. L., & Kalodner, C. R. (1990). An individualized cognitive intervention: Does it increase the efficacy of behavioral interventions for obesity? *Addictive Behaviors, 15,* 473–479.

Devlin, M. J. (2002). Pharmacological treatment of binge eating disorder. In C. G. Fairburn & K. D. Brownell (Eds.), *Eating disorders and obesity: A comprehensive handbook* (2nd ed., pp. 354–357). New York: Guilford.

Dingemans, A. E., Bruna, M. J., & Van Furth, E. F. (2002). Binge eating disorder: A review. *International Journal of Obesity, 26,* 299–307.

D'Zurilla, T. J., & Goldfried, M. R. (1971). Problem solving and behavior modification. *Journal of Abnormal Psychology, 78,* 107–126.

Fairburn, C. G. (1985). Cognitive-behavioral treatment for bulimia. In D. M. Garner & P. E. Garfinkel (Eds.), *Handbook of psychotherapy for anorexia nervosa and bulimia* (pp. 160–192). New York: Guilford.

Fairburn, C. G. (1995). *Overcoming binge eating.* New York: Guilford.

Fairburn, C. G., & Brownell, K. D. (Eds.). (2002). *Eating disorders and obesity: A comprehensive handbook* (2nd ed.). New York: Guilford.

Fairburn, C. G., Marcus, M. D., & Wilson, G. T. (1993). Cognitive-behavioral therapy for binge eating and bulimia nervosa: A comprehensive treatment manual. In C. G. Fairburn & G. T. Wilson (Eds.), *Binge eating: Nature, assessment and treatment* (pp. 361–404). New York: Guilford.

Fontaine, K. R., & Allison, D. B. (2002). Obesity and the Internet. In C. G. Fairburn & K. D. Brownell (Eds.), *Eating disorders and obesity: A comprehensive handbook* (2nd ed., pp. 609–612). New York: Guilford.

Foreyt, J. P., & Poston, W. S. C. (1998). What is the role of cognitive-behavior therapy in patient management? *Obesity Research, 6*(Suppl. 1), 18S–22S.

Foster, G. D., & Wadden, T. A. (2002). Social and psychological effects of weight loss. In C. G. Fairburn & K. D. Brownell (Eds.), *Eating disorders and obesity: A comprehensive handbook* (2nd ed., pp. 500–506). New York: Guilford.

Foster, G. D., Wadden, T. A., Vogt, R. A., & Brewer, G. (1997). What is a reasonable weight loss?: Patients' expectations and evaluations of obesity treatment outcomes. *Journal of Consulting and Clinical Psychology, 65,* 79–85.

Garrow, J. S., James, W. P. T., & Ralph, A. (Eds.). (2000). *Human nutrition and dietetics* (10th ed.). London: Harcourt.

Goldfried, M. R., & Goldfried, A. P. (1975). Cognitive change methods. In F. H. Kanfer & A. P. Goldstein (Eds.), *Helping people change* (pp. 89–116). New York: Pergamon.

Goldstein, D. J. (1992). Beneficial health effects of modest weight loss. *International Journal of Obesity, 16,* 397–415.

Grilo, C. M. (2002). Binge eating disorder. In C. G. Fairburn & K. D. Brownell (Eds.), *Eating disorders and obesity: A comprehensive handbook* (2nd ed., pp. 178–182). New York: Guilford.

Jeffery, R. W., Drewnowski, A., Epstein, L. H., Stunkard, A. J., Wilson, G. T., & Wing, R. R. (2000). Long-term maintenance of weight loss: Current status. *Health Psychology, 19,* 5–16.

Kalodner, C. R., & DeLucia, J. L. (1991). The individual and combined effects of cognitive therapy and nutrition education as additions to a behavior modification program for weight loss. *Addictive Behaviors, 16,* 255–263.

Kanders, B. S., & Blackburn, G. L. (1992). Reducing primary risk factors by therapeutic weight loss. In T. A.Wadden & T. B. VanItallie (Eds.), *Treatment of the seriously obese patient* (pp. 213–230). New York: Guilford.

Kirsch, I., Montgomery, G., & Sapirstein, G. (1995). Hypnosis as an adjunct to cognitive-behavioral psychotherapy: A meta-analysis. *Journal of Consulting and Clinical Psychology, 63,* 214–220.

Latner, J. D., Stunkard, A. J., Wilson, G. T., Jackson, M. L., Zelitch, D. S., & Labouvie, E. (2000). Effective long-term treatment of obesity: A continuing care model. *International Journal of Obesity and Related Metabolic Disorders, 24,* 893–898.

Loeb, K. L., Wilson, G. T., Gilbert, J. S., Labouvie, E. (2000). Guided and unguided self-help for binge eating. *Behaviour Research and Therapy, 38,* 259–272.

Manson, J. E., Skerrett, P. J., & Willett, W. C. (2002). Epidemiology of health risks associated with obesity. In C. G. Fairburn & K. D. Brownell (Eds.), *Eating disorders and obesity: A comprehensive handbook* (2nd ed., pp. 422–428). New York: Guilford.

Padesky, C. A. (1994). Schema change processes in cognitive therapy. *Clinical Psychology and Psychotherapy, 1,* 267–278.

Perri, M. G. (1998). The maintenance of treatment effects in the long-term management of obesity. *Clinical Psychology: Science and Practice, 5,* 526–543.

Perri, M. G. (2002). Improving maintenance in behavioral treatment. In C. G. Fairburn & K. D. Brownell (Eds.), *Eating disorders and obesity: A comprehensive handbook* (2nd ed., pp. 593–598). New York: Guilford.

Perri, M. G., & Corsica, J. A. (2002). Improving the maintenance of weight lost in behavioral treatment of obesity. In T. A. Wadden & A. J. Stunkard (Eds.), *Handbook of obesity treatment* (pp. 357–379). New York: Guilford.

Perri, M. G., McKelvey, W. F., Renjilian, D. A., Nezu, A. M., Shermer, R. L., & Viegener, B. J. (2001). Relapse prevention training and problem-solving therapy in the long-term management of obesity. *Journal of Consulting and Clinical Psychology, 69,* 722–726.

Pi-Sunyer, F. X. (2002). Medical complications of obesity in adults. In C. G. Fairburn & K. D. Brownell (Eds.), *Eating disorders and obesity: A comprehensive handbook* (2nd ed., pp. 467–472). New York: Guilford.

Rapoport, L., Clark, M., & Wardle, J. (2000). Evaluation of a modified cognitive-behavioural programme for weight management. *International Journal of Obesity, 24,* 1726–1737.

Rodin, J., Silberstein, L. R., & Striegel-Moore, R. H. (1984). Women and weight: A normative discontent. In T. B. Sonderegger (Ed.), *Nebraska symposium on motivation: Psychology and gender* (Vol. 32, pp. 267–307). Lincoln: University of Nebraska Press.

Rosen, J. C. (1997). Cognitive-behavioral body image therapy. In D. M. Garner & P. E. Garfinkel (Eds.), *Handbook of treatment for eating disorders* (pp. 188–201). New York: Guilford.

Rosen, J. C. (2002). Obesity and body image. In C. G. Fairburn & K. D. Brownell (Eds.), *Eating disorders and obesity: A comprehensive handbook* (2nd ed., pp. 399–402). New York: Guilford.

Rosen, J. C., Orasan, P., & Reiter, J. (1995). Cognitive behavior therapy for negative body image in obese women. *Behavior Therapy, 26,* 25–42.

Rössner, S. (2002). Pregnancy and weight gain. In C. G. Fairburn & K. D. Brownell (Eds.), *Eating disorders and obesity: A comprehensive handbook* (2nd ed., pp. 445–448). New York: Guilford.

Ryan, D. H., Bray, G. A., Helmcke, F., Sander, G., Volaufova, J., Greenway, F., Subramaniam, P., & Glancy, D. L. (1999). Serial echocardiographic and clinical evaluation of valvular regurgitation before, during, and after treatment with fenfluramine or dexfenfluramine and mazindol or phentermine. *Obesity Research, 7,* 313–322.

Sbrocco, T., Nedegaard, R. C., Stone, J. M., & Lewis, E. L. (1999). Behavioral choice treatment promotes continuing weight loss: Preliminary results of a cognitive-behavioral decision-based treatment for obesity. *Journal of Consulting and Clinical Psychology, 67,* 260–266.

Seidell, J. C., & Tijhuis, M. A. R. (2002). Obesity and quality of life. In C. G. Fairburn & K. D. Brownell (Eds.), *Eating disorders and obesity: A comprehensive handbook* (2nd ed., pp. 388–392). New York: Guilford.

Shafran, R. (2002). Eating disorders and the Internet. In C. G. Fairburn & K. D. Brownell (Eds.), *Eating disorders and obesity: A comprehensive handbook* (2nd ed., pp. 362–366). New York: Guilford.

Tanco, S., Linden, W., & Earle, T. (1998). Well-being and morbid obesity in women: A controlled therapy evaluation. *International Journal of Eating Disorders, 23,* 325–339.

Teasdale, J. D. (1997). The relationship between cognition and emotions: The mind-in-place in mood disorders. In D. M. Clark & C. G. Fairburn (Eds.), *Science and practice of cognitive behaviour therapy* (pp. 67–93). Oxford: Oxford University Press.

Tremblay, A., Doucet, E., Imbeault, P., Mauriege, P., Despres, J.-P., & Richard, D. (1999). Metabolic fitness in active reduced-obese individuals. *Obesity Research, 7,* 556–563.

U.S. Department of Agriculture. (1995). *Report of the dietary guidelines advisory committee on the dietary guidelines for Americans.* Washington, DC: Author.

Wadden, T. A. (1995). Characteristics of successful weight loss maintainers. In D. B. Allison & F. X. Pi-Sunyer (Eds.), *Obesity treatment: Establishing goals, improving outcomes and reviewing the research agenda* (pp. 103–111). New York: Plenum.

Wadden, T. A., & Berkowitz, R. I. (2002). Very-low-calorie-diets. In C. G. Fairburn & K. D. Brownell (Eds.), *Eating disorders and obesity: A comprehensive handbook* (2nd ed., pp. 534–538). New York: Guilford.

Wadden, T. A., & Osei, S. (2002). The treatment of obesity: An overview. In T. A. Wadden & A. J. Stunkard (Eds.), *Handbook of obesity treatment* (pp. 229–248). New York: Guilford.

Wadden, T. A., Sarwer, D. B., & Berkowitz, R. I. (1999). Behavioural treatment of the overweight patient. *Ballière's Clinical Endocrinology and Metabolism, 13,* 93–107.

Wardle, J., & Rapoport, L. (1998). Cognitive-behavioural treatment of obesity. In P. G. Kopelman & M. J. Stock (Eds.), *Clinical obesity* (pp. 409–428). Oxford: Blackwell.

Wilfley, D. E. (2002). Psychological treatment of binge eating disorder. In C. G. Fairburn & K. D. Brownell (Eds.), *Eating disorders and obesity: A comprehensive handbook* (2nd ed., pp. 350–353). New York: Guilford.

Wilfley, D. E., MacKenzie, K. R., Welch, R. R., Ayres, V. E., & Weissman, M. M. (2000). *Interpersonal psychotherapy for group.* New York: Basic Books.

Wilfley, D. E., Welch, R. R., Stein, R. I., Spurrell, E. B., Cohen, L. R., Saelens, B. E., Dounchis, J. Z., Frank, M. A., Wiseman, C. V., & Matt, G. E. (2002). A randomized comparison of group cognitive-behavioral therapy and group interpersonal psychotherapy for the treatment of overweight individuals with binge eating disorder. *Archives of General Psychiatry, 59,* 713–721.

Wilson, G. T. (1996). Acceptance and change in the treatment of eating disorders and obesity. *Behavior Therapy, 27,* 417–439.

Wilson, G. T., & Brownell, K. D. (2002). Behavioral treatment for obesity. In C. G. Fairburn & K. D. Brownell (Eds.), *Eating disorders and obesity: A comprehensive handbook* (2nd ed., pp. 524–528). New York: Guilford.

Wilson, G. T., Fairburn, C. G., & Agras, W. S. (1997). Cognitive-behavioral therapy for bulimia nervosa. In D. M. Garner & P. E. Garfinkel (Eds.), *Handbook of treatment for eating disorders* (pp. 67–93). New York: Guilford.

Wing, R. R. (1998). Behavioral approaches to the treatment of obesity. In G. A. Bray, C. Bouchard, & W. P. T. James (Eds.), *Handbook of obesity* (pp. 855–873). New York: Dekker.

Wing, R. R. (2002). Behavioral weight control. In T. A. Wadden & A. J. Stunkard (Eds.), *Handbook of obesity treatment* (pp. 301–316). New York: Guilford.

Wing, R. R., & Jeffery, R. W. (1995). Effect of modest weight loss on changes in cardiovascular risk factors: Are there differences between men and women or between weight loss and maintenance? *International Journal of Obesity, 19,* 67–73.

Wing, R. R., & Klem, M. (2002). Characteristics of successful weight maintainers. In C. G. Fairburn & K. D. Brownell (Eds.), *Eating disorders and obesity: A comprehensive handbook* (2nd ed., pp. 588–592). New York: Guilford.

Yager, J. (2001). E-mail as a therapeutic adjunct in the outpatient treatment of anorexia nervosa: Illustrative case material and discussion of the issues. *International Journal of Eating Disorders, 29,* 125–138.

Ziegler, E. E., & Filer, L. J. (Eds.). (1996). *Present knowledge in nutrition* (7th ed). Washington, DC: International Life Sciences Foundation.

Index